[redacted]

ANIMAL DOCTOR

Other books by LEON F. WHITNEY, D.V.M.

PETS
HOW TO SELECT, TRAIN, AND BREED YOUR DOG
TRAINING YOU TO TRAIN YOUR CAT
DOG PSYCHOLOGY
THE NATURAL METHOD OF DOG TRAINING
THE FARM VETERINARIAN
KEEP YOUR PIGEONS FLYING
THE COMPLETE GUIDE TO TROPICAL FISHES
DOLLARS IN DOGS
THIS IS THE COCKER SPANIEL
YOUR PUPPY
FIRST AID FOR PETS
THE COMPLETE BOOK OF CAT CARE
THE DISTEMPER COMPLEX
THE COMPLETE BOOK OF DOG CARE
ALL ABOUT GUPPIES
THE COON HUNTERS' HANDBOOK
THE RACCOON
THE COMPLETE BOOK OF HOME PET CARE
FEEDING OUR DOGS
BLOODHOUNDS AND HOW TO TRAIN THEM
HOW TO BREED DOGS
THE BASIS OF BREEDING

ANIMAL DOCTOR

The History and Practice of Veterinary Medicine

by Leon F. Whitney, D.V.M.
and George Whitney, D.V.M.

DAVID McKAY COMPANY, INC. *New York*

ANIMAL DOCTOR
The History and Practice of Veterinary Medicine

THIRD PRINTING, JUNE 1976

ISBN: 0-679-20010-X

LIBRARY OF CONGRESS CATALOG CARD NUMBER: 72-83038

MANUFACTURED IN THE UNITED STATES OF AMERICA

To All Future Veterinarians

About the Authors

ANIMAL DOCTOR was written by two animal doctors, father and son, whose combined experience covers a broad spectrum of veterinary medicine. So many young people have come to them for advice about what the profession offers, wondering whether they can find in it their life work, that the Doctors Whitney decided to put it on the line and tell it as it is. In ANIMAL DOCTOR a reader will find the subject thoroughly covered.

Dr. Leon F. Whitney started his career as a livestock farmer. Dr. George D. Whitney was born on a farm. Dr. Leon gave up farming and was for 12 years Executive Secretary of the American Eugenics Society. As a hobby he studied genetics and nutrition in dogs, work he still continues. Over 12,000 dogs have been bred in his kennels. He was a faculty member of Yale University, where he conducted research. At the age of 45 he decided to work for a Doctor of Veterinary Medicine degree, which he obtained at Auburn University. In 1941 he opened the well-known Whitney Veterinary Clinic in Orange, Connecticut. He is author of 52 books and many scientific papers.

Dr. George D. Whitney is also a graduate of Auburn University, in the class of 1943. Before attending that university he worked with his father in his scientific investigations. After graduation he spent three years in the Army during World War II doing food inspection work and as veterinarian for horses and dogs, ending this stint as a Captain. He then joined his father in the operation of the Whitney Veterinary Clinic.

The senior doctor retired to conduct research, leaving the management to "Dr. George," as he is called by the owners of the clinic's many patients.

Contents

Foreword

In presenting the information we have in this book, we tried to put ourselves in the place of a young man or woman who is considering Veterinary Medicine as a life career. What would we want to know about it? What did we once want to know ourselves? Since so many city people think of the subject as "dogs, cats and canaries," we must correct that mistaken conception.

Veterinary Medicine is an all-embracing subject with many ramifications, a fact which few people realize. All of its divisions are important for human health as well as for the health of animals. We hope we have presented a complete picture of the subject.

Our wives deserve much credit for their suggestions and help as we wrote the manuscript. We also thank Mrs. Muriel Schonfeld who edited and typed it.

Drs. Leon F. and George D. Whitney

Orange, Conn.
1973

Preface

At this time in history the challenges to the veterinary profession are tremendous. Environmental danger signals are all around us. A hundred and sixty-six species of animal life have become extinct during this century and dozens of others are threatened. Veterinarians are trained to recognize the normal and the abnormal in lower animals and must take a rigorous role in exposing problems before these problems effect mankind.

Adequate food supplies for the future must be met by containing and conquering disease and malnutrition in the food-producing animals.

With human population increasing, the over two hundred diseases communicable from lower animals to man must be watched and checked with vigilance.

Oliver Wendell Holmes wrote, "Join the action and passion of your times at peril of being judged not to have lived." In view of today's events he might have written, "Join the action and passion of our times at peril of leaving a world in which nothing lives."

History

The profession of veterinary medicine is an ancient one. Treatises written as long ago as 2500 B.C., in China and Babylonia, tell us that animal doctors were concerned with diseases of horses and buffalo, asses and oxen. The famous Code of Hammurabi, written about 1900 B.C., includes the legal fee for treating animals and the penalties for malpractice.

A little later—1800 B.C.—the Indians had veterinary hospitals. What they referred to as "the veterinary art" is what we today call veterinary medicine. An educated group of men treated mainly horses and elephants and probably oxen, if we can judge from primitive drawings. Bovine animals apparently were less important from a medical point of view, although herds of sheep were an important part of the economy.

We do know something about veterinary remedies used by the ancient Egyptian animal doctors because they left us a record of how they treated cattle and dogs.

The early Greeks made veterinary medicine a science. Hippocrates, who lived from 460 to 351 B.C., wrote about treating sick as well as healthy animals. Aristotle, whom we regard as the creator of natural science, left us writings on the treatment of sickness in animals. Both of these "natural philosophers" investigated the workings of the bodies of animals in order to increase their knowledge of human physiology. The Greeks must have been primarily concerned with doctoring horses because their name for veterinarians was *hippiatroi* ("horse doctors").

The Romans, too, were chiefly concerned with draft or riding animals. They gave those who cared for their animals' ailments the title of *veterinarius,* and a hospital where ailing animals were kept, a *veterinarium.*

With the fall of the Roman Empire, veterinary medicine, like all other sciences, went into a decline. During the Dark Ages there were few writings about animal science; nor were there many during the Renaissance, as there was in the area of human medicine. All during that period of superstition, ignorance, and cruelty, inquiry into animals' diseases were neglected. Finally, in the fifth century A.D., a Roman named Vegetius produced a book, *Artis Veterinariae* (Veterinary Art). In it he tried to dissuade his readers from beliefs in supernatural powers and influences.

In 1598, one thousand years after Vegetius' treatise, a book called *The Anatomy of the Horse* appeared, written by an Italian named Ruinii. Still there were no schools teaching veterinary medicine. The semi-skilled men called farriers (horseshoers) considered themselves able to care for a horse's ailments as well as his shoeing. How these men got their knowledge is not certain, but it was probably by the apprentice system. Thus, ignorance as well as knowledge passed from generation to generation. As recently as 1800, the veterinarian was still called a farrier.

With the increase in human population, cattle became more and more an important factor in the economy. Almost nothing was known about treating or preventing cattle diseases, with the result that losses were enormous. Herds would be decimated, be replaced, and die out again. It has been estimated that during the hundred years from 1700 to 1800, 200 million head of cattle died from epizootics (epidemics in lower animals).

Something had to be done about it. A veterinary college was established at Lyons, France. This was followed by the establishment of more colleges and by 1800 there were twenty in Europe, but none in America. During this period, many Americans were eating buffalo meat until the herds had been all but exterminated, and European cattle were imported as a source of meat. Only then was there a real need for trained veterinarians in this country.

About twenty European veterinarians came to America in the early 1800s and practiced, mostly on horses. Beyond that the farriers and self-appointed horse doctors also looked after the health of the increasingly important horse. An attempt to establish veterinary schools in Boston and Philadelphia failed, but the New York College of Veterinary Surgeons did produce some graduates in 1867.

After the Civil War, a number of schools sprang up, mostly to teach horse-doctoring, and by 1927 more than 11,000 men had been graduated. These schools were two- or three-year institutions. When the internal combustion engine was developed the need for horses became less and less. Many of the veterinary schools soon closed and today none of these "horse-doctor" institutions remains, although a few of their older graduates still practice. The first modern College of Veterinary Medicine was opened at Iowa State in 1879.

ANIMAL DOCTOR

1

What Is Veterinary Medicine?

Anyone considering the profession of veterinary medicine as a career needs to know all the facts he can get. The dictionary defines veterinary medicine as "That branch of medicine which concerns itself with the study, prevention, and treatment of animal diseases." The definition omits an important concern of the profession: the prevention of the spread of diseases from animal to man.

If you come from an urban area you may think that the practice of veterinary medicine means caring only for dogs, cats, and pets in general. A dean of one of the veterinary colleges showed us a breakdown of 1,700 applications received by that school: only a minority of the 1,700 were from young men from farms. The great majority were from men and women in cities. Over 500 of the applicants were living in New York City. Many of these applicants will remain in the city, treating poodles and parakeets, but others will head for the country, where they will work with food-producing animals.

A great many who have consulted us about veterinary medicine as a profession expect their work to be confined to companion animals. In the city they have owned pets of various kinds and have accompanied them to local veterinary establishments and have seen the treatment given them. Some have worked in local veterinary hospitals either in their spare time or have spent entire summers working there because they want to pursue the profession as a life's work.

On the other hand, there are young people from farms who have no knowledge of how a city veterinary hospital is run. They have a completely different idea of veterinary medicine. Some may have accompanied veterinarians on their calls and been impressed with the wonderful service that can be offered in saving the lives of animals and preventing disease.

Because there are so many aspects to the profession of veterinary medicine you must understand at least the main ones. If you do attend a veterinary school, you will have to learn them all and you will have to be prepared to work in any one of many fields.

Veterinary medicine can be described as the study of the normal and abnormal in lower animals. When one considers the number of lower animals, this is a broad field. For a student to learn even the normal anatomy of all lower animals would be an impossibility, and therefore specialization is necessary.

In our country the profession of veterinary medicine came into being to fulfill the need of caring for work animals, and later food animals, and more recently, companion animals. Research in all areas followed as the need increased. During the past thirty years research results have been pouring into the professional journals at an ever-increasing rate, particularly as concerns the problems in lower animals that are similar to those in man. In a large percentage of man's ailments we have a similar problem in some lower animal.

The versatility of veterinary medicine may best be explained by examining the duties of the veterinarian in a few specific fields.

Are you interested in horse flesh? The work of the race track veterinarian is quite different from the work of the veterinarian caring for pleasure horses or working on Thoroughbred breeding farms where animals may be worth from \$5,000 to \$50,000 or more. Practitioners for bovine animals may have 90 percent beef cattle to work with or may work with dairy animals almost exclusively. The researcher may be in charge of sending animals up in rockets for an Air Force project or may be studying leukemia-like diseases in cats. The companion-animal veterinarian may specialize in cats or in ophthalmology and have practitioners refer cases to him or her from a large surrounding area. The mixed-animal practitioner may, in addition to working with all animals, spend a few hours a week inspecting carcasses at a local slaughterhouse. The areas of endeavor are endless: nutritionists working with animal-food farmers, fur-ranchers, or companies that process food for animals, or as pathologists examining the remains of all sorts of creatures to find what diseases are present. This work may save countless others.

We hear more and more about plans for veterinary schools, where, after two years of study, a student will decide on an area of specialization, and for the last two years of his training will do intensive study in that area. Such specialization may necessitate changes in state board examinations.

Veterinarians regard their profession as one of the most worthwhile of all professions. The senior author was, for many years, on the faculty of the Yale Medical School where he did research, and he knows from his close association with many physicians and fellow research workers how much there is also to be said for human medicine. In fact, some of his veterinary education was a year's study at Yale where he took seven courses. He could have chosen to be a physician, but he was determined to obtain a veterinary degree and is glad he did. He would do it again.

But we are not acting as missionaries trying to lure you into veterinary medicine. Before you have finished this book you will learn that this is a demanding profession.

The American Veterinary Medical Association divides the field into the following classes and, on the basis of a verification survey conducted for the AVMA in 1970 for the United States, here is the total number of men and women in each class.

Large animal	1,416
Mixed practice	7,424
Small animal	5,758
Other classes	3,790
Public health	360
Regulatory veterinary medicine	1,443
Military veterinary medicine	833
Unknown	970

This study was broken down by states. The ratio of general practitioners to small-animal specialists is much smaller in heavily populated urban areas than in more sparsely populated rural areas. Vermont has only seven small-animal specialists and forty-three veterinarians who are engaged in mixed practice, for Vermont is a rural state in which the number of dairy cattle is about equal to the human population.

California reports 355 in mixed and 1,058 in companion-animal practice.

New York, 337 in mixed and 471 in companion-animal practice.

Wisconsin, 284 in mixed and 65 in small animal practice.

You will be interested in knowing what these different classifications encompass and we will try in the following chapters to give you an unvarnished, factual picture of veterinary medicine.

We have talked with dozens of people from cities and suburbs who love animals and want to devote their lives to keeping them healthy. Do they really know what kind of profession it is? To young people who have an erroneous idea of veterinary medicine, we suggest they take a trip to one of the big hog farms, or to a dairy farm, or beef cattle ranch, and after they spend some time looking around the farms to return and then we will talk.

"Oh! That's not my idea of a vet's job," some people may say.

"What is your idea of it?" And we learn that the person owned a number of pets or some baby chicks and loved them all. We further learn that these people may have observed only the workings of a city animal hospital.

While there are 5,758 veterinarians who specialize in companion-animal health, this segment of the profession is less important on the basis of its *economic worth* to the country as compared to the huge field of farm animal care.

Dogs and cats are not regarded by Congress as domestic animals. Except for those animals used in research, our government cannot appropriate money to help them as it does to help cattle, swine, poultry, sheep, and horses.

Because the farm dog is an economic asset to stockmen, some work has been done for them by Uncle Sam. But not because they were companions or guards.

The eighteen states which have established veterinary colleges did so to train animal doctors to keep farm animals healthy because these creatures are tremendous economic assets to the country.

To help you appreciate the enormity of the farm animal field and the opportunity for service in it, consider the fact that probably 30,000,000 young pigs die of disease every year. This is a third of all of those born. Over 235,000,000 chickens and 7,200,000 turkeys die of disease annually. So do 250,000 horses. Of the other four-legged animals saved to weaning age, 1,500,000 cattle, 2,500,000 calves, 4,000,000 sheep and lambs, and 10,500,000 hogs all die from diseases each year. An estimate of the value of the annual losses of livestock from diseases and parasites is upwards of $2,500,000,000.

The opportunities are tremendous for study and action in the parasite field alone. Over 300 kinds of internal parasites are known to take a toll of livestock. This reduces the possible gross from livestock and poultry over $400,000,000 a year. Insect pests cause a loss of over $500,000,000 a year.

We must always keep in mind there are many kinds of values. Money is one. Friendship is another, and to us is of much higher value.

While the individual companion-animal owner values his or her animal sentimentally, the stockman values his economically. Veterinarians are called on to treat all kinds of animals, but federal and state governments appropriate funds chiefly for *farm animal health*. So, the emphasis of veterinary medicine must be on large animals, with companion-animal health subordinate.

Not that the companion animal field isn't important; it is. If anyone doubts it, just remember that the sale of pet foods in 1970 has passed the $1,300,000,000 mark. It is estimated that besides this huge amount spent on pet foods over $1,000,000,000 of food for humans in fed to pets annually. Dogs eat one-twentieth as much food as the human population.

There are 35,000,000 or more dogs and probably an equal number of cats and the specialists who try to keep them healthy are truly an economic asset to the country, but not so considered by authorities.

Try writing to the dean of admissions of any veterinary college. Say you are a city person who has always loved animals. You have kept rabbits and hamsters and your family has always had a dog. Even if your marks are excellent, you almost certainly will not be accepted.

But suppose you could say, "I've grown up on a stock farm. We have 600 head of White Face cattle. We market about two carloads of hogs annually. I hope you find my marks acceptable as well as the enclosed letters of recommendation." The dean can scarcely turn down such an applicant.

And then there's the in-between applicant. He may write: "I hope the fact that I was reared in a suburb won't be held against me. All my life I've handled animals. As Dr. Smith's letter will tell you, I have worked in his hospital in my free time and have ridden with him on his outcalls to assist him in caring for farm animals. Every summer I've worked on a different kind of stock farm to learn all I could about animals. I enclose letters from the men who employed me." Such a student is wanted by the veterinary colleges.

The last two applicants talk the language of the stockman.

They speak of "200 *head* of cattle" or "120 *head* of hogs." They are unlikely to say "200 cows" or "120 pigs." They know how to handle manure forks and the sight and feeling of blood doesn't bother them. They have seen death many times and, while it makes an impression every time it is witnessed, it doesn't throw them. They most likely have visited slaughterhouses and have perhaps seen living animals converted into human food. They realize that all those millions of head of beef cattle and hogs and lambs are raised for food and though they become inured to death, they do not necessarily lose the sensitivity in their own temperaments.

We advise that every student who loves pets and wants to become a veterinarian pay a visit to a big packinghouse and spend some time observing. Watch the sheep being led up the long incline by the Judas goat who turns around and goes back down again to lead another pen of sheep to their death. Watch the almost mechanical precision with which hogs are butchered. See how the packer uses "every part but the squeal." Observe the cattle being converted into beef. Talk with the veterinarians who spend their time inspecting carcasses in order to protect the human population from possible disease. And as you watch, remember that your education will include a required course in meat inspection.

Go to a dairy farm and watch its operation from the time the cows are turned out to pasture in the morning until they come in, in the late afternoon, each going to its own stanchion. Watch the milking process, remembering that it is part of the veterinarian's job to insure that the milk doesn't contaminate human beings with disease as it surely would were the veterinary safeguards removed.

Find an opportunity to watch one or more veterinarians at work. Ride with one on his outcalls or watch him give treatments in his hospital. What to him may be routine may seem to you to border on the miraculous.

What might you see on such trips?

A farmer goes to the pasture with his dog to drive his cows in to be milked. He is shocked to find lying about the pasture perhaps a dozen or more of his cows all but unconscious. Then he remembers that only yesterday he vowed he would cut down and burn all those wild cherry sprouts along the fence row. He races back to his house and phones the "vet." The doctor is not home but his wife calls him on the two-way radio and in ten minutes the doctor is in the pasture giving intravenous injections. Every cow still able to breathe is saved. All he had to do was to give a drug which neutralized the cyanide which the cherry leaves in the cow's stomach were pouring into the blood. That done, he and the farmer get the cattle into the barn and pour glucose into them, because glucose causes the action to reverse the chemical reaction and thus detoxify the stomach contents.

There are many other dramatic treatments such as the giving of emetics which empty poisoned dogs' stomachs, surgical procedures equivalent in every way to those the medical physician performs.

We hope you haven't the usual movie image of the typical veterinarian. In many of the Westerns the veterinarian is a dirty, messy old man, almost always with a cigar butt in his mouth. His close companion is the stable boy, and the two of them doze in the hay beside the sick horse until daylight when the horse raises its head, cured. What a sorry image! Today, the veterinarian is a skilled professional. He wears clean uniforms when he calls on his patients, and he is so busy he seldom has time to spend the night with one patient.

It may be a surprise to learn that every veterinary college

has a goodly number of older men in attendance. There are those who have not found their jobs satisfying and, now finding it financially possible, have decided to do what they have always wanted to do—become veterinarians.

The colleges know that these men are often among their most successful graduates. Among our friends is one of the top large animal veterinarians in the West. He is a natural with horses and cattle. He was a rodeo rider for years until, at the age of thirty-eight, he went to college. Others who later became veterinarians were once a top bacteriologist at Harvard; an executive in a telephone company; manager of a pet store; a poultry specialist; and a high school principal.

Some of the advantages this vocation offers are:

- The great satisfaction in helping the animals one treats and thereby helping the owners.
- The prevention of the spread of over two hundred diseases transmissable from lower animals to man.
- Through investigation and observation of lower animals one can directly benefit mankind.
- Security; you aren't likely to lose your job.
- You are your own boss.
- You need not commute; you can live in or near your office or hospital.
- Good pay.

Some of the disadvantages, depending on the field of choice are:

- Your time is seldom your own. This is a confining profession. It is difficult to plan and carry out vacations. Your nights are often disturbed by emergencies.
- This is a strenuous profession, so one needs to be physically strong.

- The feeling of helplessness in dealing with certain diseases, especially the virus-caused group.
- Emotional upsets, caused by having to break the news about the death of an animal to its owner.

2

The Large-Animal Practice

According to the last agricultural census, there were in the United States in 1972, 120,000,000 cattle, 20,000,000 sheep, 57,000,000 swine, and 8,000,000 horses and mules. There were 70,000,000 small pet animals. There are approximately 22,000 veterinarians in the United States to guard the health of those animals other than poultry. This comes out to one veterinarian for every 13,409 four-legged animal. This number includes veterinarians employed either by the Federal government or various state governments who aid the Practitioners. Almost all of their work is done on farms and not in veterinary hospitals. A small number of veterinarians specialize only in the practice of horses and some are permanently attached to race tracks. At one time, even within our lifetime, the greater part of large-animal veterinary work *was* concerned with horses as indicated by textbooks in veterinary schools which featured the horse, while other species were almost incidental. However, the number of horses and mules dropped from 24,211,000 in 1910 to 3,000,000 in 1960. Millions of animals were killed and their flesh canned for dog food. Some meat was sent abroad to countries where horsemeat is commonly eaten by human beings.

The 21,211,000 horses which disappeared were almost all work animals. Then something happened and the horses began to increase in numbers. In twelve years, 5,000,000 were added to the horse population.

The horse today is not so much an economic asset or a food animal as he is a means of giving pleasure. Some horses are used in the woods in lumbering operations, some are ridden by cowboys in herding, and many still are used on farms where the land is too steep for agricultural machinery. There are also race horses and horses bred for shows and exhibitions, trained for jumping, for hunting, for hacking, for polo and rodeos. Thousands of ponies give children and some adults hours of riding pleasure. Veterinarians are called less frequently to administer to work horses than to pleasure horses.

Nearly all of the large-animal veterinarians occasionally take care of dogs, cats, and other companion animals which are brought to them, but they cannot be considered specialists in the field. Some live many miles, fifty or a hundred, from the next veterinarian and in such sparsely settled country, there are few companion animals for them to care for anyway.

Just what do these large-animal doctors do to earn their living? The work they do necessitates their having sound constitutions, for a lot of it is hard physical work. Much of it is surgery, a great deal is vaccination and testing. And remember, cattle and hogs are not picked up easily and handled. They are driven into chutes where they are restrained by mechanical means.

A typical large-animal veterinarian has an office, a small hospital or at least a few cages, and an operating table, a laboratory, X-ray, and a secretary, who is often his wife. His car is fully equipped with the necessary instruments and essential drugs, an insulated cold box to preserve vaccines and serums. There is a telephone in the car so the doctor can keep in communication with his home base. From day to day his work is a constant adventure. But overall, the large-animal man:

1. Makes calls to care for individual ailing animals.

2. Performs necessary operations where economically feasible. This is determined by the animal's value as a breeding specimen, or its market value based on its weight and condition. In other words, the animal is worth what the owner can sell it for. If the animal needs an operation, a farmer or rancher will weigh its sales value against the veterinarian's fee and the trouble he will have in caring for the animal after the operation is performed. Then he makes his decision.

3. Tests cattle. This entails determining whether all the cattle of a given area are free from tuberculosis and from brucellosis (Bang's disease). The first fact is determined by injecting some tuberculin within the skin and returning three days later to "read" the results. To test for Bang's disease, blood must be drawn from a vein and sent to the state laboratory. Undulant fever (it's called Bang's disease in cattle) is a serious disease in man, as anyone who has had it will tell you. The senior author caught it from a goat on which he was working and was sick for many months. Cattle found to be infected with Bang's disease are condemned.

A good illustration of how the veterinarian prevents human illness is seen in the buffalo herd of 600 animals on the Crow

Indian Reservation in the mountains of Montana. These buffalo were the property of the government. Each year the Indians were permitted to shoot 10 percent of the herd to keep it small enough for the 16-mile-square enclosure. After each reduction of the herd, many Indians became sick with undulant fever. Veterinarians were employed to take blood samples of the 60 buffalo shot one year. The tubes of blood were sent to the state laboratory where it was found that a high percentage of the animals had undulent fever. So high, in fact, that the entire herd was ordered destroyed. They were replaced with calves from the Yellowstone herd, which were first vaccinated against the disease.

Goats must be tested also. The disease from goats in human beings is called *Brucella melitensus;* it is also called Mediterranean fever. Swine have the disease too, *Brucella suis,* which produces an especially severe disease in humans. Dogs have *Brucella canis,* which also affects man.

4. He tries to prevent the inception or the spread of diseases. He may be called to immunize a herd of swine against hog cholera or other swine diseases. He may immunize against a disease called "black leg" in cattle. If a rancher or stockman is planning to ship carloads of cattle to market, he asks his animal doctor to inject them to prevent shipping fever, an ailment which often makes them unmarketable. Their price would naturally drop if they had to be put aside to recover, since their weight would be considerably less.

5. The large-animal veterinarian is particularly concerned with keeping down parasites in his clients' animals. If he lives in the south, this is an acute problem. The farther north he lives, the less serious it becomes. Thus, he may be called to deworm a whole flock of 600 head of sheep. Perhaps a herd of hogs is dewormed another day, or a herd of horses. The

veterinarian responds to all calls, whether everyday work or emergency.

6. He must be able to give advice on husbandry. One of the most essential and rewarding segments of the veterinary field is that of reproduction. Most farm animals must increase if they are to be economic assets. A cow should produce a calf every year or she will not continue to produce milk. The breeding sows on a hog farm or the beef cattle cows on a ranch must all reproduce to supply the owners with the pigs or calves which, when grown, constitute the market crop. The brood mares on a Kentucky bluegrass farm are not there as ornaments; they must produce foals which will be sold or raised for racing or riding; the sheep in a flock are not kept just for their wool but for the lamb chop which is their most valuable asset.

If anything is wrong which lowers or destroys fertility, it becomes of the greatest concern. Discovering the cause becomes the veterinarian's task. He may save an owner hundreds of times the cost of his fee by his diagnosis.

Another aspect of reproduction is the treatment of those diseases which prevent it. One is contagious abortion, or Bang's disease mentioned above. Other diseases are treated with drugs and biologics.

Statistics show that over one-tenth of all dairy cows fail to expel the placenta and the membranes which have enveloped the calves during pregnancy. These must be removed by hand. The average large-animal veterinarian receives many calls to perform this task.

Difficult births require his attendance just as obstetricians are needed at the birth of babies. A great many cows or mares or ewes or sows have trouble. The offspring may be twisted and need to be placed in a normal birth position before it can be born. Some young are too large for the mother to pass naturally. Nearly every farm boy or girl has watched or perhaps assisted the veterinarian as he helped the female give birth to her offspring.

A new generation every year for almost all livestock, except work horses, is practically a must for livestock men the world over. Naturally, therefore, the veterinarian is needed to insure the success of breeding programs. You may have watched a veterinarian don a rubber glove and sleeve and reach inside a cow to feel the condition of her ovaries. He may have been called by the owner who reports that the cow hasn't come in "heat" for too long a time. The doctor feels a "lump" on the ovary called a corpus luteum, exerts a special kind of pressure with his trained fingers, feels the "lump" pop out of the ovary. The "lump" was preventing her coming in "heat." Now she will soon be ready for breeding and probably will become pregnant.

Artificial insemination is often practiced for economic and other reasons. A goodly number of veterinarians specialize in this work. In livestock areas throughout the United States one finds barns in which there will be one each of five or more breeds of bulls: Jersey, Guernsey, Holstein, Brown Swiss, Santa Gertruda, Ayreshire, Hereford, Aberdeen Angus. Farmers whose cows are in "heat" phone the center which sends an inseminator who inserts a tube into the cow and forces a little diluted bull semen into the uterus. Most of the time the cow becomes pregnant and the farmer is saved the cost and danger of keeping his own bull.

Moreover, the quality of the bulls is generally much higher than any one farmer can afford. Before any bull is bought for breeding purposes, he must have proved that his calves will tend to be superior, so most of the bulls have some age and require special handling.

Artificial insemination is practiced with many species of farm animals. Today semen is sent by mail and used successfully in this highly specialized work.

7. Besides these functions, every large-animal veterinarian assists Federal veterinarians in preventive and emergency work. A suspicion that foot-and-mouth disease has broken out means a drastic quarantine, and the local professional must enforce it.

The work of the large-animal veterinarian is similar to that of a public health officer. Not only does he enrich livestock owners but he guards mankind against the diseases which farm animals could, without his careful work, spread to man. He must know about these dangers. He may live in a state where rabies is prevalent. A suspicious dog is captured and incarcerated in the local pound or in one of the doctor's cages. The animal must be watched and all local animals immunized, the public alerted, the livestock men told to watch for strange behavior in their stock, for who knows what creatures the dog may have bitten. One rabies scare terrifies any community and the head man in the affair is the veterinarian.

8. A new kind of veterinary medicine is evolving in which when you are graduated you may become involved by choice. This is called by many names, such as *contract work*. The doctor enters into an agreement with a stockman and agrees to help him with all his animal problems for a year. He helps with nutritional problems, fertility problems, growth, parasite, marketing problems. One veterinarian can handle only a limited number of animals and that number is dependent upon the population of the ranches and farms of his clients. Indeed, there are quite a number of ranches so large that they each employ a veterinarian full time.

As stated at the beginning of this chapter, there are about 13,409 animals for each veterinarian. But this is really only an average. Among the 22,000 veterinarians there are many specialists. Some work only at race tracks where all the horses they care for and test for attempted doping may not number over 500. These specialists reduce the number who must watch over the health of much larger numbers of livestock. Riding with a veterinarian in Wyoming, you may pass a tremendous flock of sheep, later a ranch where 30,000 head of cattle graze, then a large hog farm. All of these, and many more, are his patients. So you see, there are some animal doctors who have many more animals to guard than others have, or choose to have.

One more occupation of hundreds of veterinarians is that of passing on animal health in stockyards. All over our country there are sales stockyards. To them, once or twice a week, the stock is brought to be sold. Too bad that so few of us have had the opportunity of watching this important segment of American life in action. Some yards move but a few hundred animals, while the turnover of others runs into the thousands. Huge trucks transport animals in and out.

Some stock will be sold for slaughter but a great many sold for fattening. A large part of the American corn crop is sold for livestock feed. Farmers buy the range-grown cattle and feed them corn which increases their weight to more value than the corn would bring if sold at commodity prices. The stock is in pens, and the cattle or hogs are driven out onto a scale and then into a pen around which sit livestock buyers who bid on them.

When the livestock is sold they go into other pens and are loaded into trucks. These often are two-story affairs which carry great loads. But before any single head of livestock moves out, it is inspected by the veterinary inspector. He may be a very busy man. On hot summer days, heat prostration in stock is common. Not only must he watch the health of animals but act as an humane officer as well. Almost all of these inspectors are local men who contract to do this work on a yearly basis, which adds materially to their income.

There are several examples of veterinary discoveries and the applications of them have proved of enormous significance. In addition to having reduced the reservoir of human tuberculosis by the constant testing of farm animals, Texas fever, also called tick fever, comes to mind. This was a devastating disease until it was learned that the bite of a tick named *Boopholis* caused it. Thousands of cattle in the south where ticks thrived died of the disease during the hot summer months. Those that recovered were debilitated and their value greatly reduced.

The disease was spread by shipments of cattle infested with the ticks which dropped off and infected other cattle. When veterinarians discovered that ticks were responsible, a widespread dipping order was introduced. The cattle were driven through huge vats that contained poisons. This killed the ticks on the cattle. Then it was learned that if there were no cattle living in an area, no matter how badly the area might be infested with ticks, for fifteen months, all the ticks died out for want of animals to feed upon. All wild deer had to be exterminated because the ticks feed on all undulates.

Today, due to the meticulous attention of veterinarians, Texas fever is practically extinct, with the exception of certain Indian Reservations where diseased wild deer and ticks infect cattle. Constant vigilance must be exerted to prevent new outbreaks along the borders of the reservations.

3

The Mixed Practice

While one learns in college to be an all-around veterinarian, the graduate is free to practice in the field of his or her choice. Perhaps it is logical to expect that the city-bred veterinarian will, after graduation, practice in the city. But this does not necessarily hold. Actually, many of them elect to settle into mixed practices. No one can be completely unmindful of finances and it is obvious that, where country-practice overhead is so small compared with opening a city hospital, the large-animal part of mixed practice offers great opportunities.

There are over 7,400 veterinarians who list themselves as "Mixed-Practice Veterinarians." These doctors, as the name suggests, take care of all species, not specializing in either large or companion animals. Some work out of hospitals where more than one veterinarian is in attendance and where one of the doctors is always at home to see clients with companion animals while the other is on the road attending to farm animals. Or both may see companion animals and operate during rush hours and make farm calls at other times.

The majority of mixed-practice veterinarians work singly from their cars or station wagons when making outcalls on farm animals and work at companion-animal surgery when convenient and are in their offices in connection with their hospitals to receive clients and treat animals presented at stated hours. The clients learn that these hours may be interrupted by emergency calls from farms. However, they are often farmers themselves who understand how serious such emergencies may be and find no fault with the doctor if he has to leave them for an emergency call. He may ask the companion-animal owner to leave the animal in a cage to be treated when he returns. Such treatment is not acceptable in a city hospital. The same applies to suburban veterinarians who try to work at mixed practices; in time most of them learn that the two kinds don't mix and so they limit their practices to small-animal work as residential areas take over farmland. Witness the fact that there are now 5,758 who look after only companion animals, whereas in 1940 there were only 11,000 veterinarians in all areas of the profession.

There are millions of dogs and many other companion animals on farms. In many of our states every dog must, by law, be vaccinated against rabies. This means hours of work. Some country veterinarians advertize that they will hold a "rabies clinic." A steady stream of dog owners appears and each dog goes home vaccinated and with a tag attached to his collar. Farmers and their sons are often hunters and their hunting dogs need attention as well as their stock dogs and guard dogs. The mixed-practice veterinarian devotes a good share of his time to dogs, but his fees are almost never as high for that service as are the fees of city veterinarians. This is because of lower veterinary overhead, and the farmer does tend to regard his dogs and cats as economic rather than sentimental assets. And in passing, we should note that the farmer's dogs are on the whole better, sounder dogs temperamentally. He won't stand for defects in temperament which the city dog owner coddles and often perpetuates.

4

The Companion-Animal Practice

This is our field, although it wasn't always. We feel that our services have helped to make thousands of persons happy. We try to make the owning of companion animals as enjoyable as possible. Now, while we have stressed that this division of the profession is not economically comparable in importance to the great field of large-animal practice, you must know that with over 35,000,000 dogs and the same number or more of cats, their health must be guarded too. There are only 5,758 of us in this field, mostly practicing in cities and in suburbs. We care for 70,000,000 animals, chiefly dogs and cats with sentimental value, compared with 8,840 general and large-animal practitioners who guard the health of 214,000,000 farm animals whose value is mostly economic.

The term "companion"-animal specialist is preferred over the term "pet"-animal specialist because there are so many animals which are not pets at all. Among the dog population are several million hunting dogs: hounds, among which are beagles, foxhounds and coonhounds: bird dogs, such as pointers, setters, spaniels and retrievers. Their owners do not think of them as pets. Some farm dogs are taken to suburban veterinarians and these are not pets but rather stock dogs or guard dogs.

True, some of the dog breeds are physically larger than some livestock animals. Lambs are often kept as real pets, so there is some overlapping in terms, but companion-animal specialist is the preferred term.

In this context the term specialist is used loosely because the companion-animal physician and the large-animal physician are the last of the general practitioners in any of the healing arts. We find true specialists developing in the profession such as ophthalmologists, orthopedists, radiologists, and surgeons.

At one time city veterinary practice was almost exclusively horse practice. Back in 1900, there were 24,211,000 horses and mules, and the human population of our country was 75,994,575. This was one horse for every 3.1 persons. Small wonder that veterinary medicine was mostly "horse practice" then. By 1930, the human population had grown to 122,775,046, but horses and mules numbered 16,683,000, a ratio of one for seven people. Today we have 8,000,000 horses and 203,000,000 people: one horse for every twenty-five people. No wonder the emphasis is no longer on horses. The city horses which did all the hauling trucks do today, are almost all gone. The old horse doctor has gone too. Some veterinarians say that the dog took the veterinarian out of the stable and put him into the living room, but actually the sophistication of the entire profession brought about its present place in society.

It is our impression that at present rates charged by large-animal practitioners, their practices are as remunerative as other practices. Nevertheless, there are those who prefer the small-animal work. Work in this field consists of:

1. *Surgery:* This involves a wide variety of operations. Accident cases are numerous and they often entail setting bones. Skin surgery is naturally part of it too. There is frequent surgery to repair lacerations from dozens of causes. Chains around the neck often wear through the skin. It is surprising all the woe which human beings inadvertently inflict on their pets. Cut feet often need attention. Bird shot must frequently be extracted. And in the north, removing of porcupine quills is not uncommon.

Of all the individual operations, ovariohysterectomy is the most common. The average number in most busy hospitals is about five a day, and more should be done to prevent thousands of unwanted puppies and kittens.

Litters of puppies are presented for ear cropping. Some states permit the operation by anyone, but some permit only veterinarians to perform it. In England, this operation is considered inhumane and is outlawed. Many animal physicians consider it immoral to inflict pain just to please the vanity of an owner. This is our feeling. Tail docking is less objectionable.

Bone setting and the preliminary X-raying figure high on the list of operations. Considerable skill is required to insure that the animal's leg is set so that in time he will be normal. Bones are sometimes maintained in place with stainless steel pins inserted in their marrow. Many ingenious mechanical devices may be used to hold the broken legs in their normal positions.

Cancer surgery is high on the list of procedures. Joint surgery to correct traumatic and hereditary defects are common.

Urinary calculi (stones), kidney surgery, intestinal surgery and exploratory surgery are commonly performed. Amputations are less common. Dentistry in all forms is an everyday occurrence.

As the number of toy dogs among the dog population increases, the number of Caesarean operations needed increases too. The breeders of some breeds such as Boston terriers and Chihuahuas often expect that every bitch may need to give birth by surgery and are happily surprised when they do not. In these instances, the dogs' doctors can advise their clients to help cut down the misery which indiscriminate matings of their dogs can bring. They can urge them not to breed bitches which do not whelp naturally. A knowledge of genetics is a valuable asset to every veterinarian.

2. *Diagnosis:* Will Rogers once said if he ever became ill he would go to a veterinarian because you don't have to tell him what's wrong with you. Using the symptoms and the information often extracted from the owner and the massive information obtained from laboratory tests tempered with education and experience leads to a diagnosis. It is true detective work. Many tests cannot be performed in most veterinary hospitals and so experts are consulted for results—pathologists, toxicologists, and biochemists.

With companion animals living closely with man, the diseases communicable from them to man must be controlled as expeditiously as possible. Not infrequently the public must be educated to a potential disease problem. In this area of public health, the companion-animal veterinarian takes the leading role.

3. *Immunization:* Time was when every dog was expected to have distemper and all we could do was to hope he would live through it. At that time, distemper could have been any of a dozen different diseases or combinations of them. On one

occasion, we had 90 of our own dogs with the disease and buried 75 of them. At one time the term distemper embraced Carré's disease (true distemper), hardpad disease, canine hepatitis, and leptospirosis, to name four of the most important diseases in that complex of years ago. Dogs can be given a program of vaccinations to protect them all their lives from contracting these diseases. Such a program has a high percentage of success. Leptospirosis is communicable to man, so the veterinarian acts once again as a public health agent.

Rabies is another disease against which dogs need protection. Every species is susceptible. By immunizing dogs in states where cases have been known to occur, the human and dog population are protected against its ravages. In Georgia, veterinarians of both small and large animal practices vaccinate over 200,000 dogs a year. Immunizations constitute quite a considerable part of the companion-animal doctor's practice.

4. *Treatment or Therapy:* The knowledge that an animal has been properly immunized usually, but not always, rules out those diseases in a diagnosis. Once a diagnosis has been established, treatment begins.

The owner of a sick companion animal wants either to have the veterinarian treat the animal in the hospital or to treat his animal himself at home. Naturally there are some diseases which no one wants to have at home. Distemper is one, a protracted disease which necessitates a lot of care. A cat with ringworm may spread it to all the members of the family before the animal is cured. We know of one innocent-looking long-haired kitten which actually closed an entire schoolroom. Some of the children had their heads shaved. The kitten was taken to school by its owner, it was handled by the children and spread the disease. A dog with leptospirosos is dangerous to keep at home. There are many diseases which the veterinarian is called upon to treat in his hospital. It constitutes a considerable portion of his practice but nowhere nearly as large a share as it was before effective vaccines were developed.

5. *Husbandry Advice:* Considerable time must be assigned to the education of the new animal owner concerning diet, training, grooming, the innoculation program and personality problems, to name a few. Advice on breeding and whelping is often sought. Most of us learn from animals of our own, knowing that firsthand experience is necessary as well as formal education.

6. *Treating the Owner:* It has been said that the companion-animal veterinarian does more good for the mental health of our land than many times the human psychiatrists, and we are inclined to agree. Untold numbers of lonely people have little to look forward to in their lives other than the affection shared by them and their animal friends.

A good bedside manner is an asset to any companion-animal doctor. The word *prognosis* means *outcome*. With experience the practitioner is able to neither overemphasize nor to minimize the prognosis. He has a high batting average in predicting the outcome of each case presented. With a better and better educated public the time of explaining the rationale of a course of treatment is usually appreciated. It engenders the confidence so important in the cooperation of the owner in home treatments.

All the divisions of companion-animal veterinary medicine are important. There are others, but most of the work can be classified into the six fields just covered. In several states, the associations of veterinarians have agreed that it is unethical to board pets, and some feel that it is unprofessional to groom them. All are against advertizing excepting modestly in the telephone yellow pages. No veterinarian should publicly offer boarding and grooming facilities. And these are indeed profitable because one of the doctor's assistants can be, and usually is, delegated to do that work.

The American Veterinary Medical Association has adopted a strict code of ethics embraced by most state associations. Nevertheless, a few veterinarians run pet shops as adjuncts of their practices. Some have stores where they sell animal foods, leashes, harnesses, toys, books, and what not. The person who is particular about being professional opposes such enterprises and most state associations are antagonistic to them. If you have been associated in your spare time with a city veterinarian who operated such an institution, don't count on establishing one yourself because it is probable that all of the veterinarians will have given up everything but ethical practice by the happy time when you are granted your veterinary degree.

The companion-animal division of veterinary medicine is a profession of what the economists call "diminishing returns." The income is greatest when the practice consists of a small hospital, sometimes even a store, and one assistant. When, with the growth of practice, other veterinarians and assistants are added, the owner often makes less net income because of the greater overhead. This fact is acceptable and progressive veterinarians constantly add more and better services to their establishments.

Statistics show that the more doctors, the less the caseload of each becomes. Usually the heavily endowed institutions are those which employ several doctors. They may feel less incentive than the man who runs his own establishment and therefore may do less work each day. Some of the institutions have to ask every year for public donations. They do much free work but the actual figures indicate the doctors in them seldom turn out as much work as the man who works for himself. Many veterinarians average about forty cases per day. One large, publicly endowed veterinary hospital averaged nineteen and another only twelve.

You can expect to make many good friends through having treated beloved animals, but to the practitioner, the satisfaction of the job well done in saving an animal is the highest reward.

Too many clients take for granted the wonders of the antibiotics and other new drugs. They have not known the situation before these substances were made available and so they do not —cannot—appreciate that today animals survive diseases where a generation ago there was scant hope for them. But because they expect so much, few clients can accept the fact these drugs do not destroy viruses. So when an animal dies of a virus disease, the owner often becomes angry at what seems to be the doctor's ineptitude. A simple explanation is necessary with every case to prevent such a judgment.

Then there's the client who takes his animal to you and says, "Fix him up, Doc. He's the only one we have and we don't want anything to happen to him." These people are accustomed to driving their cars to a garage and telling the mechanic, "Put in a new clutch" or "Fix the carburetor." Life isn't like that.

These same people don't take Grandma to the hospital and say, "Fix her up, Doc. She's the only grandmother we have." So is it any wonder that a lot of explanations are due? All this comes under the heading of treating the client. Part of it is educating clients, and if it is done with tact and kindness and with a good bedside manner, it wins many clients and friends for the profession.

Much of what we have said concerns dogs. The cases in most practices of other species of animals rank small in proportion. All the statistical estimates show that cats are as abundant as dogs and we think they are much more numerous, because most of the estimates relate only to cats in homes or on farms. Few accountings take the feral cats into consideration. There certainly are dozens of times as many of these gone-wild creatures running about in woodlands adjacent to farms and suburbs as there are dogs. Wild dogs are a rarity. One game warden trapped over 500 cats one year and all far from homes. A game-bird farm superintendent trapped 450 in one year—all homeless cats. But we are concerned with the well-cared-for cats. If there are as many as there are dogs, then cats either have many fewer sicknesses and ailments than do dogs or the owners do not present them for necessary treatment.

Cat owners, however, value their pets as highly as do dog owners and expect to pay as much for their medical attention as do the dog owners. There are great satisfactions for the veterinarian in caring for cats, especially because many of their viral diseases respond to supportive treatment.

A goodly part of cat work consists of neutering and immunization. Very few cat owners can tolerate the odor of a tomcat and, knowing that castration ends it, they almost all have the operation performed. Cat fights frequently result in infected wounds which require treatment. Ear mites are found infecting cats' ears in a large percentage of cases.

In the United States one of our national problems is to further reduce the prevalence of rabies. Rabies is the concern of veterinarians in most areas of endeavor, as well as of public health officials. When a suspicious case is observed, it is the local veterinarian who is called on to handle the animal. When the animal is quarantined, it is often in a veterinary hospital.

In 1971, 235 rabid dogs were identified. Skunks accounted for 46 percent and foxes for 15 percent of the cases. There was a total of 4,392 cases among all animals, but with each year a slight decrease among dogs has been recorded. When any rabid animal bites a cow or horse, it may constitute a heavy loss to the owner. Undoubtedly there are many cases which die undiagnosed. Rabid cats behave so differently from rabid dogs that they are often undetected, yet they bite livestock and transmit the disease. When a human being is bitten, he is given treatment that is very painful. Over 30,000 persons bitten annually are given this treatment, which has no doubt reduced the number of deaths from rabies—from nine in 1956 to about one per year since them. Veterinary control programs are credited with the reduction.

Some small-animal veterinarians have made such enviable reputations in treating cage birds that a fair part of their practice consists of curing their ailments by drugs or surgery. Yes, parakeets especially, develop tumors, some benign and others malignant, and surgery of a delicate type often prolongs their lives many years. People who have spent hundreds of hours teaching a parakeet to talk are naturally solicitous for the bird's welfare. Indirectly, the animal physician who has contributed to the well-being of a lower animal has also contributed to the well-being of its owner.

5

The Food Inspection Veterinarian

The trained veterinary food inspector is an important public health protector. At first thought a prospective veterinarian might say, "I wouldn't want that job. It's too messy." It really isn't.

It seems incredible that actually over 800 carcasses are inspected every minute of every working day—at least 100,-000,000 every year, or 70,000,000,000 pounds of red meat and meat products. People want meat and the veterinary inspector's job is to see to it that they get it clean and free of diseases and parasites. In some carcasses only certain parts have to be condemed. Thus, in 1954, 2,400,000 calf and cattle livers were condemned; about 13 percent of all cattle slaughtered had diseased livers. Federal inspectors condemned over 100,000 swine for fifty different causes. Parts of more than 1,600,000 were condemned. Every day a total of

1,000,000 pounds of meat and meat products are condemned.

There are poultry inspectors who, with their assistants, study live and dressed poultry for diseases. Human beings can contract tuberculosis from chickens, psittacosis from ducks.

There is the stockyard veterinarian who inspects every steer, cow, calf, hog, sheep, and goat unloaded into pens to be sold at auction.

Then, in every packinghouse, small or large, a veterinary protector of public health observes first the animals to be slaughtered and then the carcasses. He may slice through a lymph gland, feel a little grating with his trained fingers, and perhaps condemn a $250 carcass to be made into fertilizer, thus protecting you and me from illness.

He has his own office at the plant, he writes reports, and, because he works in a large establishment, directs his assistants. He advances quite rapidly, has a comfortable salary to live on, has time for leisure and a later pension. He is a specialist.

The food inspector does a very good job. Without careful food inspection think of the cases of food poisoning there would be! True, after food is cooked it is safe, but how about all the people who handle meat up until the time it is cooked? This includes the housewife who prepares the raw meat and fish. Two generations ago, women very frequently were infected with huge tapeworms (some as long as seventeen feet), but men rarely were. Why? A food inspector learned that because women often tasted an uncooked mixture of lake fish and spices to be sure it was properly flavored, they ingested cysts which the worm larvae had formed in the fish muscles and the cysts developed into tapeworms. The men ate only the cooked product and cooking had killed the cysts.

The word of the veterinary meat inspector is law. If he says, "tank the carcass," it is not used for human food. It may be heat treated in a huge sealed tank under pressure and the ground-up meat scrap used for animal food, but rest assured it no longer has any infecting organism in it.

He forces the buyers of livestock to buy only healthy animals. We can assure you from experience that were it not for his ever alert guardianship, unscrupulous dealers would be butchering diseased creatures and selling them to the public. Even under present conditions, dealers are buying day-old calves, killing them, and lying about their age. The law says a calf to be vealed—killed and sold as veal—must be at least six weeks old. Anything younger is called bob veal. Untrained lay inspectors, who are tolerated in some local communities, are sometimes bribed to pass bob veal as edible so that thousands of day-old calves are butchered and their flesh sold as veal.

Goat meat is frequently sold as lamb and much more would be, without veterinary inspection. There really isn't much difference between the flesh of a young, well-grown kid goat and that of a lamb, but the public likes to know what it is eating. Veterinarians are taught in college some simple differences and they can quickly tell which is which.

Older animals are naturally more likely to have chronic diseases than are the younger, so the inspector is extra careful in scrutinizing their carcasses. Especially those of old bulls, because bull beef makes the best hamburg—best flavor. Of course, as roasts and steaks you could scarcely chew it, but hamburgers are made of *ground* beef. Why must the inspector be so careful about inspecting old bull beef? Because so many hamburger cooks only brown the outside leaving the center nearly raw. Parasite cysts and germs of many kinds aren't heated enough to be killed, so if uninspected beef were eaten as partially cooked hamburgers, imagine the disease such beef could spread.

Hogs spread trichinosis. Of course no one today should ever have it after all the warnings about the dire results of not thoroughly cooking pork. But despite those warnings, thousands of cases are reported every year. And every hog carcass gets the closest inspection from the veterinarian. He condemns many, but some do escape his detection. A few days before writing this, we heard a man in a restaurant order "pork chops, rare." And Jersey pork chops at that, at least so the menu advertised. A great many Jersey pork chops are made from garbage-fed hogs. It is mostly from garbage—particularly *uncooked* garbage—that pigs and hogs get infected with trichinosis. A law requires that garbage that is fed to hogs is supposed to be cooked. One of the veterinarian's jobs is to see that it *is* cooked. But he can't be around to kill the millions of rats that eat the garbage in the hog pens along with the hogs. The hogs often snap a trichina-infested rat and eat it, becoming infected themselves.

Having trichinosis is a painful experience. Knowing that one is helping to cut down on the incidence of it and many other diseases in his fellow human beings is one of the smaller satisfactions enjoyed by the veterinary food inspector.

Not all food inspection is done by graduate veterinarians. The Federal Meat Inspection Program is carried out by about 900 veterinarians and 3,700 trained inspectors. Another Federal service called the Poultry Division of the Consumer and Marketing Service of the United States Department of Agriculture employs 525 veterinarians and 2,000 inspectors who are not graduates.

The cost to the public is between 50 and 60 cents per person a year. It's the cheapest health insurance in the land.

6

The Research Veterinarian

The veterinary scientific research worker, like nearly all other researchers, knows that his greatest reward will come from the realization that he has added to the world's knowledge. He is paid enough to support a family but his prospects of getting rich are not great.

Veterinarians are constantly being reminded that a large part of the science underlying their profession has been gained by students in other fields who used dogs, cats, and other species in their work. Scientists conducting nutrition experiments have supplied a great deal of information essential to animal health. Research surgeons have established the basis for human surgery through their research with laboratory animals, including dogs and cats. Their findings have been of enormous help to veterinarians.

In some cases, veterinarians have discovered facts and

methods which human physicians find essential. Bone pinning —which now helps human beings with broken bones to get well faster—began with a veterinarian's attempt to discover a better way to set bones. Some gland transplantation and an understanding of the effects of some drugs had their origin in the work of veterinarians.

Today, original research by veterinarians for veterinarians is going ahead full steam. Some of it is conducted by practitioners who carry it on as a sideline to their practice, and some by veterinarians who are employed by commercial companies. Of course there are many working for the Federal Government who are among the most astute and useful scientists.

In his book *An Introduction to Science,* J. Arthur Thompson sets down what he thinks are the distinctive features of the scientific mood. He says: "The scientific mood is especially marked by a passion for facts, by cautiousness of statement, by clearness of vision, and by a sense of the interrelatedness of things. It is contrasted with the emotional or artistic mood, and with the practical mood, but the three form a kind of trinity (of knowing, feeling, and doing) which should be unified in every normal life."

If you feel that you have these qualities, together with a love of inquiry, you should put them to work at veterinary research.

We have been both practitioners and researchers. The satisfaction we've felt from our modest research achievements far outweighs that which we have experienced from practice. In practice you can help a limited number of animals, in research what you learn may help millions.

"What do you get out of it?" What all researchers receive —*satisfaction* and a reasonable remuneration.

Those research men who have given us methods of immunization against virus and bacterial disease have conferred enormous benefits on our animals. In fact, the basic principle in the immunization of dogs against one disease—distemper—is the same used in the famous Salk polio vaccine.

Where can the veterinary researcher find employment? There are universities who are glad to have them. A goodly number are employed by the Federal Government, many large commercial companies, and the military.

The universities may employ the veterinarians to keep the hundreds or thousands of monkeys, dogs, cats, and rodents they use in research in proper health. The animal pathologist in particular contributes much in the way of knowledge gained from their research.

If "the past is prelude to the future," let's look at some of the research done by members of the profession.

Suppose you had been a veterinarian in the state of Kansas in 1912, you would have doctored many horses because at that time horses had not been replaced by machinery. Summer came and all of a sudden you received so many calls from horse owners that you could scarcely keep up with the demands on your time. In 1912, 40,000 horses died from among the 160,000 that contracted sleeping sickness. But that was before veterinarians learned how to control the disease. This turned into a public health problem because human beings were affected, too. When children were stung by the infected mosquitoes which spread the disease among horses, half of them died.

When a disease has affected a large number of animals, the situation is described as an *epizootic*. The equivalent term in the case of human beings is an *epidemic*. When a disease strikes or threatens to spread, we quarantine human beings, but the veterinary method often has to be destruction of the infected herds, not only of the sick animals. By resorting to this method, some enormously destructive diseases have been conquered by veterinarians.

Another discovery also comes to mind which has had widespread consequences for mankind as well as for his farm animals. Undulant fever is a human disease which, as those who have been ailing with it will tell you, is a most debilitating and grave disease. It causes chills and fever and lasts for many months. We contract it from animals in several ways, but principally from drinking raw milk and in handling raw meat.

In cattle and swine it is called Bangs disease and is so serious that all of the animals known to be affected are destroyed. The states pay local veterinarians to draw blood from cattle, send the samples to the state laboratory where it is studied, and if the animal from which the sample is taken is positive in the test—has the disease—that animal is condemned, removed from the herd and destroyed. Thousands of beautiful animals are condemned annually.

Probably you never heard that it was veterinary research which brought to the attention of researchers in human medicine the fact that blood organisms transmitted by insects could cause diseases. In 1888, Theobold Smith discovered the protozoan parasite in cattle blood that was responsible for tick fever. Sixty-five thousand dollars was spent on this classic research into animal diseases. Every year since the discovery was put to work eliminating tick fever in cattle, it has saved farmers over $60,000,000—*every year*. But better still, this discovery opened the door to the discoveries which led to the control of malaria, yellow fever, typhus, and bubonic plague in human beings.

When hog cholera struck in the last century, farmers were certain that hogs would become all but extinct on farms, but research demonstrated that a filterable virus was responsible, that immunization was possible. Patiently veterinary scientists

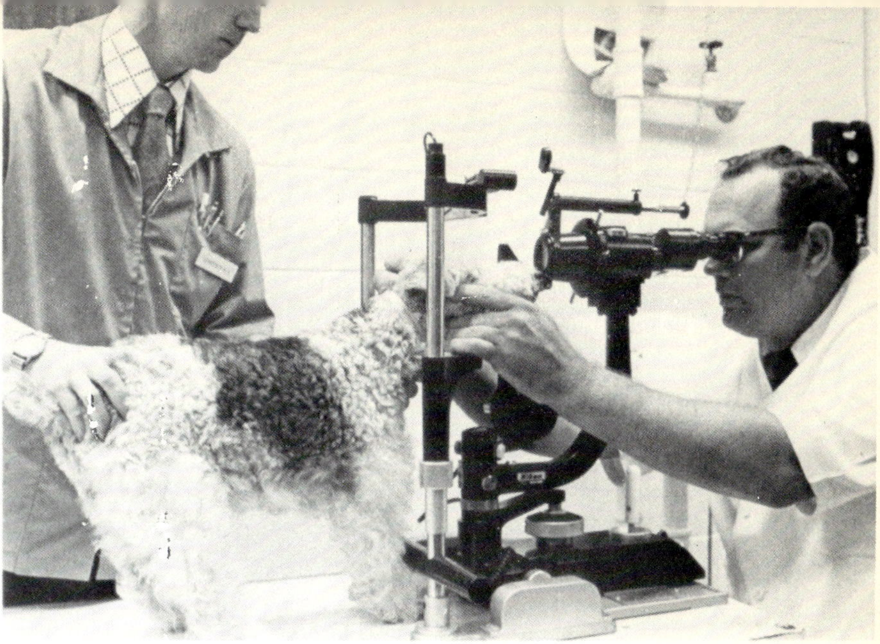

A veterinarian studies a wirehaired fox terrier for visual defects.

These puppies will be weaned and vaccinated.

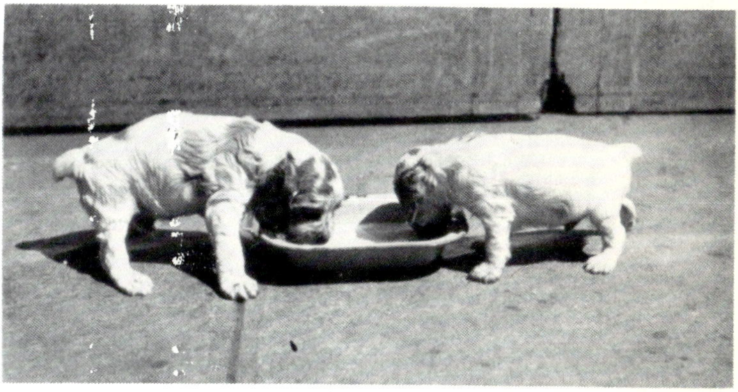

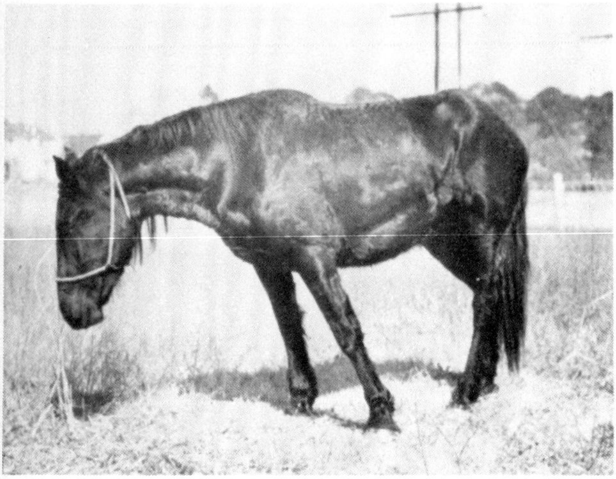

Vaccination could have saved this horse from death by encephalomyelitis transmitted to him by mosquito bites.

Healthy, happy hogs that are well cared for.

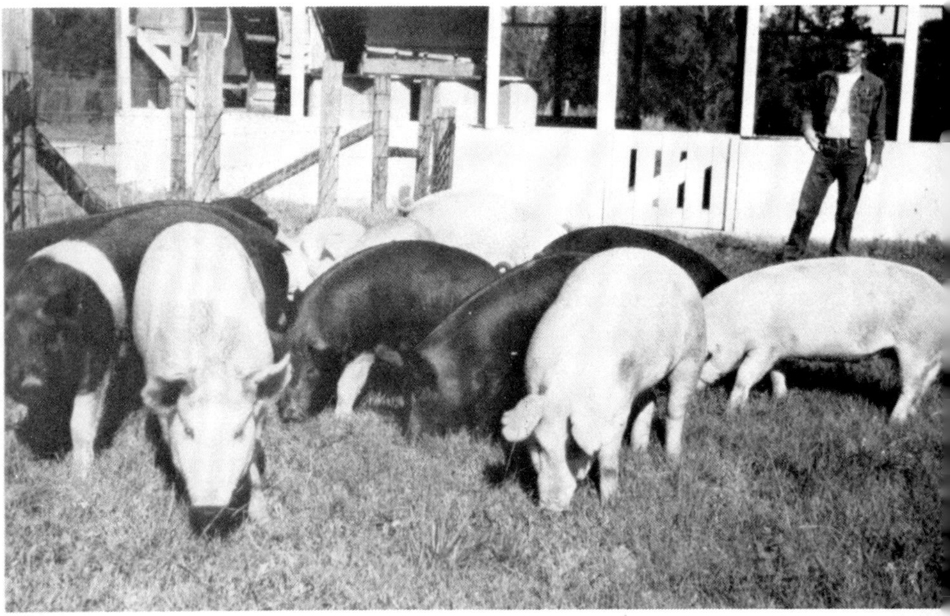

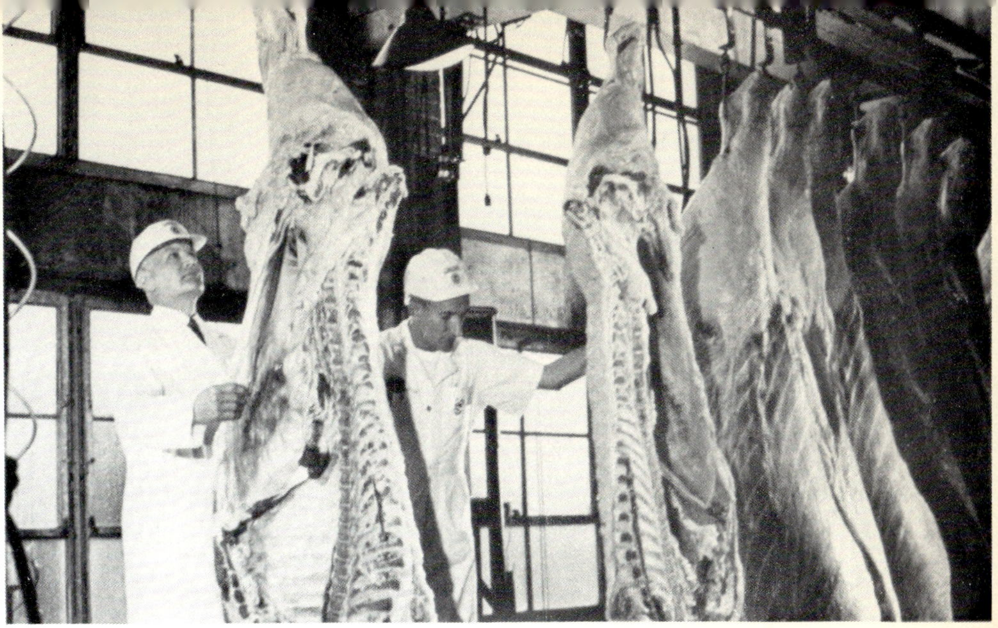

Courtesy of USDA

All beef carcasses for public use must be inspected by veterinarians.

Food inspectors guard us against eating contaminated meat.

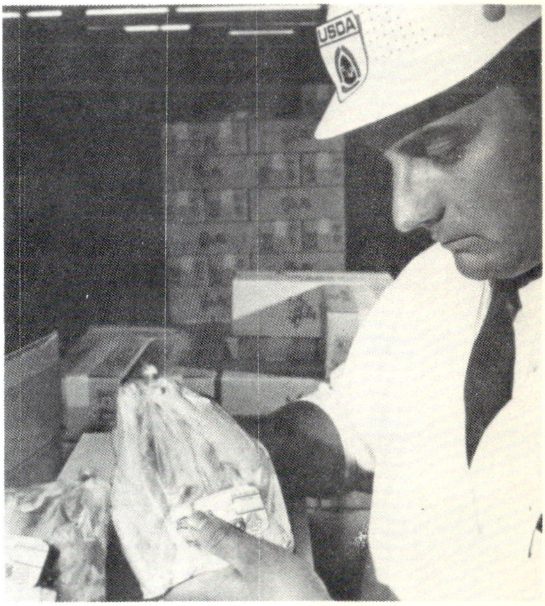

Courtesy of USDA

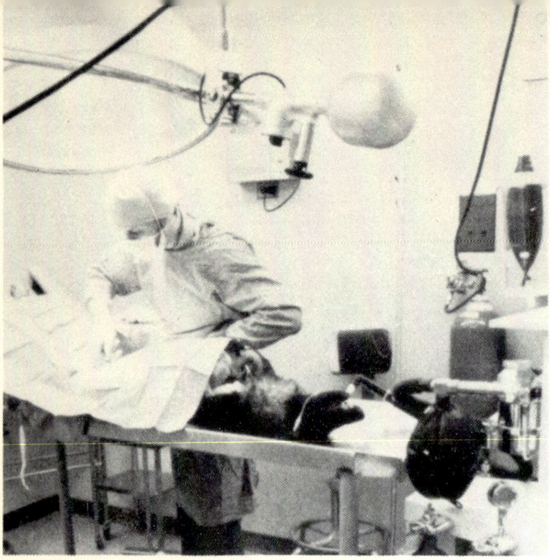

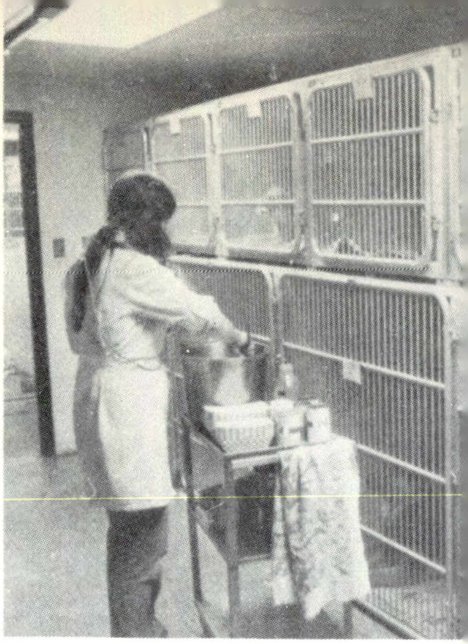

Upper left A veterinary surgeon's equipment is sterile and of the highest quality.

Upper right Each animal will be fed separately according to his needs.

Drugs are used extensively on animals. Veterinary hospitals must be well stocked.

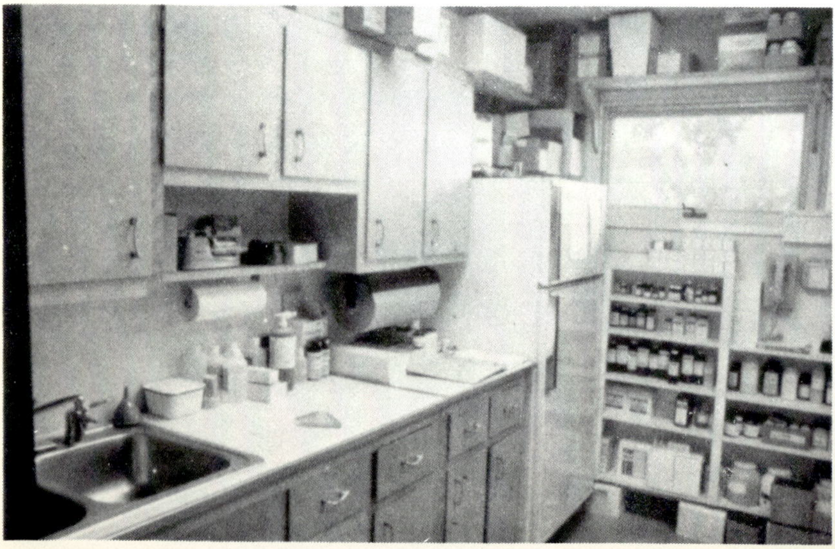

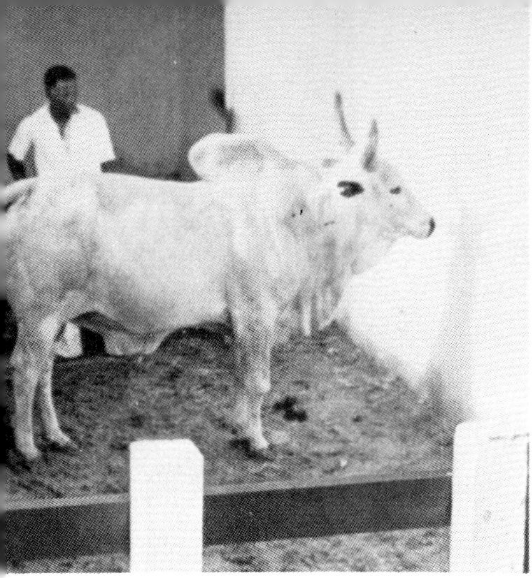

A fine, specially selected Brahma bull used to produce hybrids.

Until recently, a horse with a broken leg would have been shot. This mule's leg has been saved by setting it in a sling.

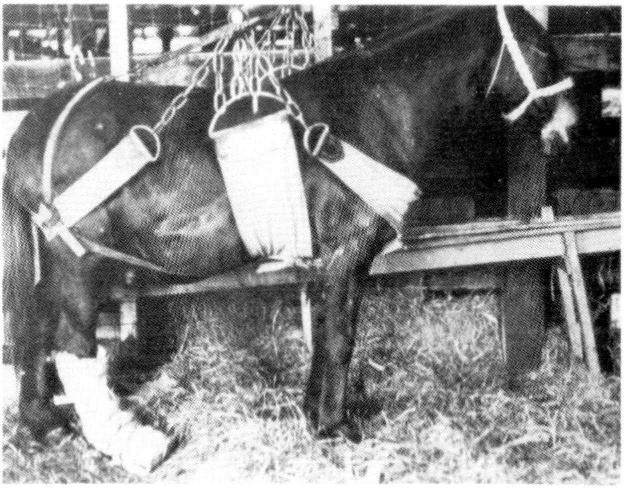

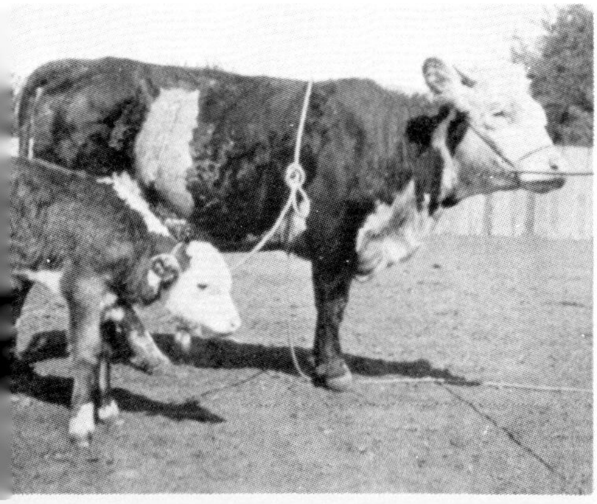

A Hereford cow and calf that were saved by a Cesarean operation.

The doctor's patients . . .

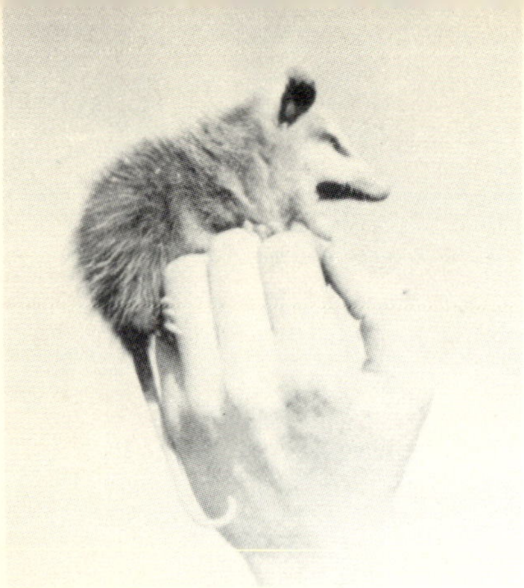

Possum

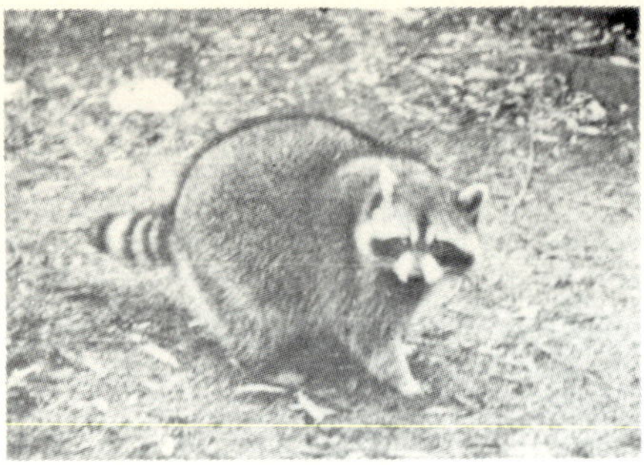

Raccoon

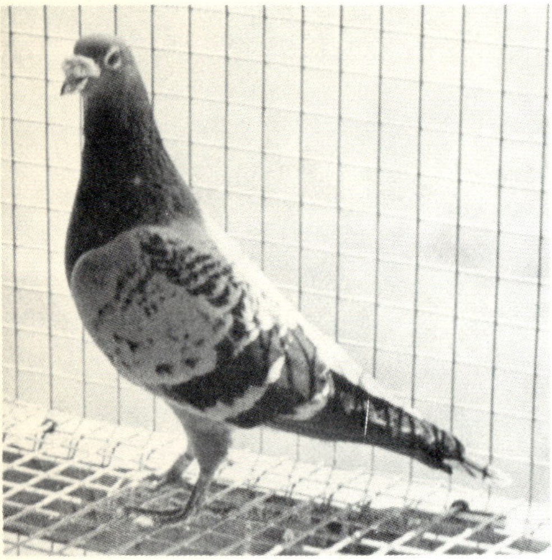

Pigeon

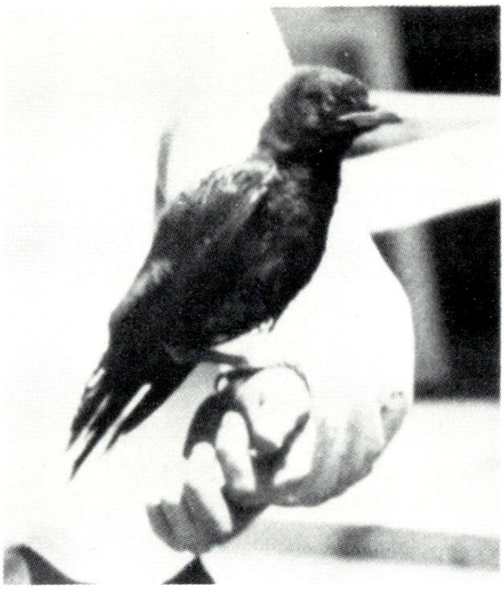

Baby crow

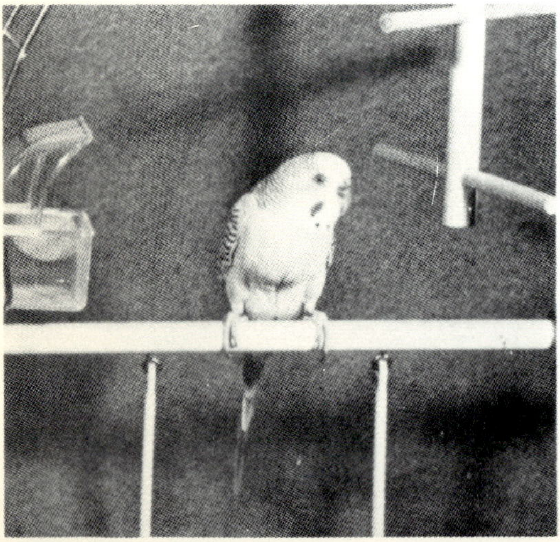

Parakeet

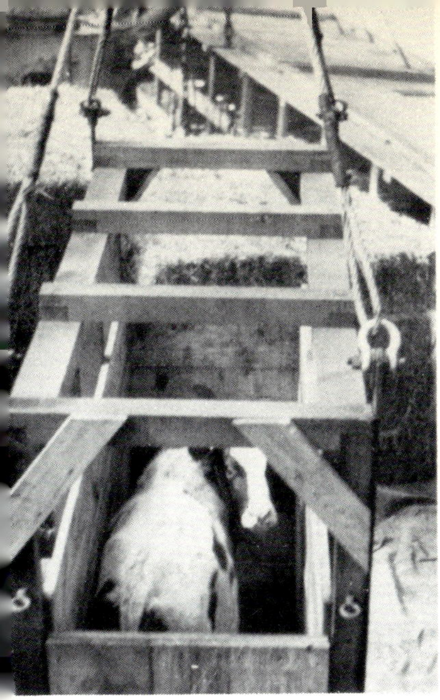

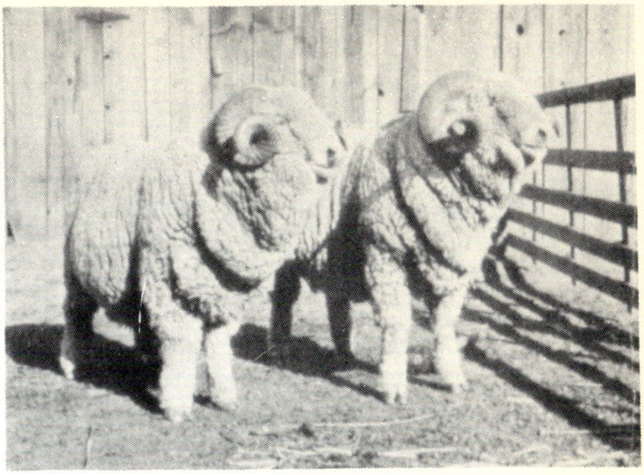

Upper right Breeding rams must be kept separate from the ewes of a flock. These Rambouillets will be turned out with the ewes in the early fall.

Upper left Veterinarians supervise the safe loading of cattle onto ships.

The veterinarian will draw a blood sample from the buffalo cow. The sample will be studied for Bang's disease before the meat is judged safe for consumption.

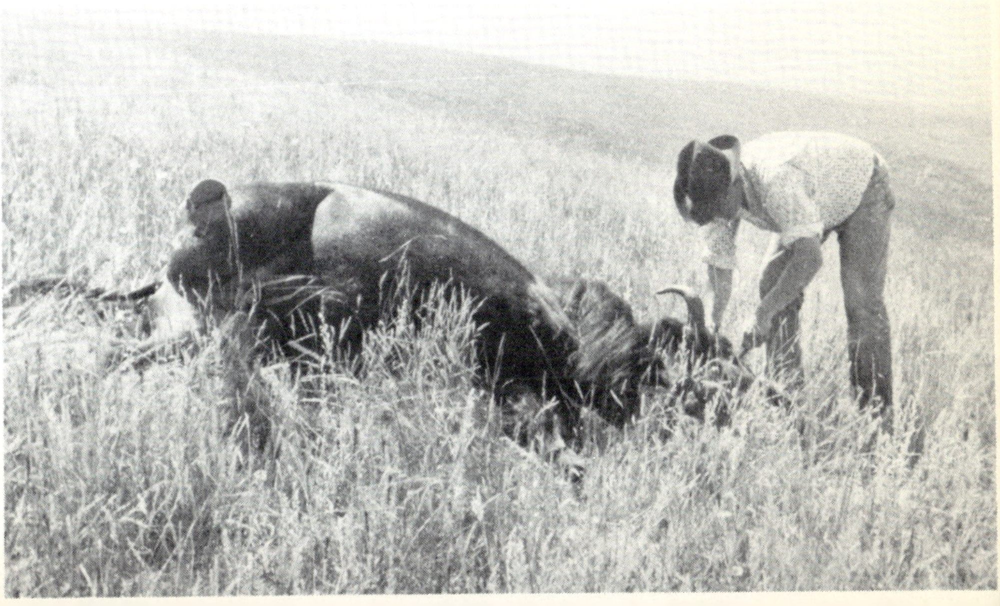

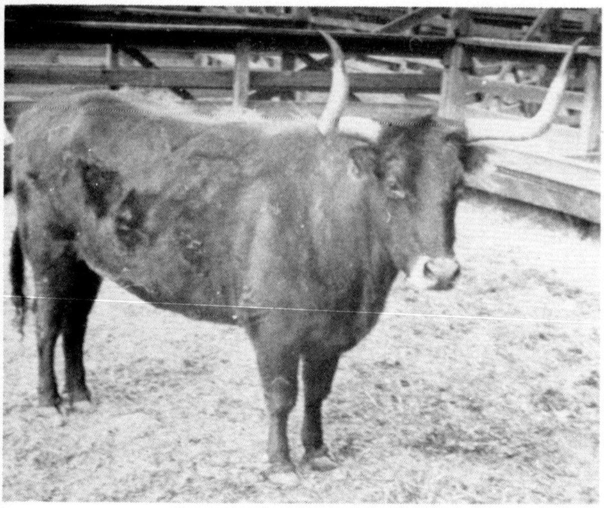

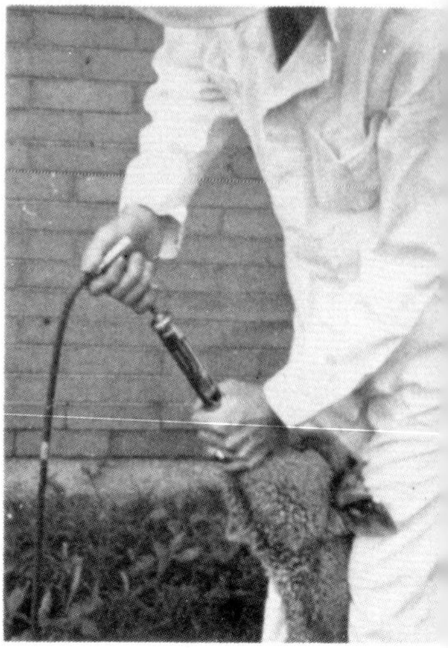

Upper left This Texas Longhorn, which will be thoroughly tested, is the last of the Will Rogers herd.

Upper right A veterinarian doses a ewe with liquid medicine.

An animal doctor treats his patients with the same instruments employed in a hospital for humans.

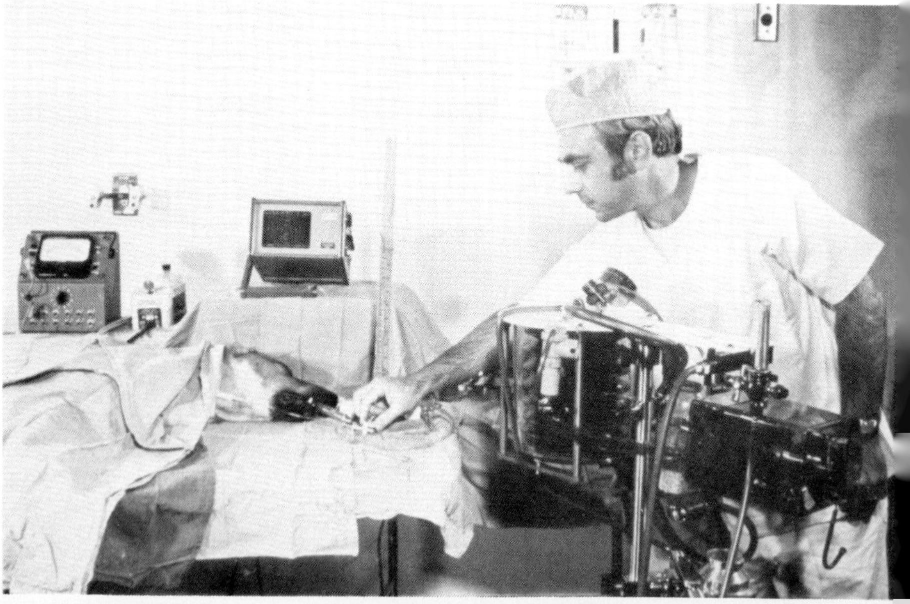

produced the vaccine and actually worked out several different methods, until today the disease is no longer dreaded.

Our Federal Government and states spend upward of $150,000,000 annually keeping tuberculosis in cattle in check. They are fighting parasites in livestock, parasites which exact a toll of over $1,000,000,000 a year. If you become a veterinarian, perhaps you can devise methods to cut this toll drastically.

What kinds of research are there to follow? The variety is enormous. One may choose to work in the discovery of antibiotics either within the confines of a laboratory, or making trips to search for strange soils from which to extract them.

Or perhaps another brand of research would take one "into the field," by which is meant working actively with animals. By studying what environmental factors destroyed 166 species of animals in the last 2,000 years and what factors threaten dozens more, one could contribute a great deal to mankind.

Suppose you have discovered or have heard about a chemical—perhaps a biological drug—which when injected into a cow with a retained placenta would cause her to expel it naturally instead of its being necessary for a veterinarian to remove it manually. You want to see whether it will really work, so you must travel extensively to many cattle farms, injecting cows and then return to these farms to determine the effectiveness.

Then again you may have discovered a treatment for mastitis (infected udder) you think is better than any yet tried, so you must first obtain the cooperation of farmers who will notify you of any suspicion that a cow is infected, whereupon you go to the farms and try the treatment.

Perhaps you have discovered a promising treatment for skin infection in dogs. You must accumulate data to test whether it is superior or inferior to accepted treatments. This means you must find dogs to treat and perhaps use a standard remedy on one side, and your own on the other side of each dog.

Or, you have indications that a certain drug can actually penetrate body cells and kill virus particles without damaging the cells. Animals must be assembled, infected with some virus diseases and half of them treated with the drug, the untreated half being the controls.

Challenges of the Future

Foot-and-mouth disease *is* dreaded. Despite all precautions by quarantining, inspection and sanitation, the disease has managed to bypass these defenses six times since 1900. Large numbers of cattle must be destroyed each time. Our veterinarians were sent to Mexico and England to help control devastating epizootics in those countries. The Mexican government had imported some Brahma cattle to cross with Mexican cattle. They were quarantined on Sacrificio Island off Vera Cruz. Natives sneaked cows to the island on rafts at night and bred them to the Brahma bulls. Soon, foot-and-mouth disease spread like wildfire over Mexico. The cost of control ran to $134,500,000 for the United States just to keep it south of the border and help the Mexicans eliminate it. Where will it strike again? The guardians against it are the veterinarians.

While there are about 13,875,000 dairy cows within our nation's boundaries, one inconspicuous disease alone accounts for an animal loss to our farmers of over $500,000,000. It has been estimated that if one-third of those cows could be replaced with cows without the disease, the amount of milk produced would be enormous. Or to put it another way, we could get along with many fewer cows because we would have enough milk. The disease is called *mastitis,* an infection of the udder.

Veterinarians are not only helping to overcome this defect in the cows but they are carrying out tests to determine where it exists. Many farmers do not realize what the disease is doing to their stock and pocketbooks.

Commerical organizations, foundations, Uncle Sam, all employ research veterinarians; and every man in the work seems to be leading a rewarding existence.

7

The Teaching Veterinarian

The eighteen veterinary colleges have approximately three hundred faculty members. A few of the professors are retired practitioners, most of them are young men who love teaching and, as in the case of the research man, derive much satisfaction from the kind of life that teaching affords. Some combine research with their teaching.

Each faculty member concentrates on his specialty as do the professors in a medical college. Some teach pathology, some microbiology, physiology, others medicine and pharmacology, anatomy, surgery, to name a few. One man heads the large-animal section, specializing in the teaching of diseases of large animals, another in small-animal diseases and care.

In the preveterinary courses which all students are required to take, nutrition is often taught after organic and physiological chemistry. Now a majority of veterinarians are being consulted by their clients on feeding, and especially the mixing of drugs with food, to promote growth rates and prevent disease. Consequently the subject of nutrition is coming to have a more important place in the veterinary curriculum and is being taught as one of the principal veterinary courses.

Except for pathology, the poultry inspector has been almost outside of the veterinary profession, but more and more, this subject of poultry is becoming an important one in the veterinary curriculum and teaching specialists are in demand.

Veterinary medicine, in some ways, is a more difficult subject to learn than human medicine. The human physician must know about only one species, *homo sapiens;* the veterinarian must know well all of the species with which his profession deals. He must know the anatomical differences. This in itself presents a challenge, because the differences are so great. A member of the ox family has four important sections to its stomach, one of which holds about fifty gallons. In contrast, the single stomach of an average-size dog which, while enormously expandable, usually is called on to hold no more than a quart or two.

A chicken has a gizzard, a horse has no gallbladder, a cow or bull has a small intestine 147 feet long, a horse has one that measures 72 feet. Cattle, sheep, goats have no upper incisor teeth; other species have them. The differences in the reproductive systems are especially diverse. The lengths of gestation periods run from sixty-one days to eleven months. The mare has two teats and produces one colt, usually; the sow has a dozen or more teats and produces nine to fifteen pigs.

Physiological differences too, as one might expect, vary from species to species. The dog gulps his food. He has very little of the starch-digesting enzyme in his saliva, while ox family members not only chew the food well but belch it up and chew it again, to mention only a few of dozens of differences which might be cited as examples.

Even the drug tolerances and methods of administration vary from species to species. One can use phenol on a dog, but it may kill a cat. Horses can't vomit, or if they try, the vomitus runs out through their noses; but dogs, cats and hogs vomit freely. So, the veterinarian must be careful about the drugs he administers. What may cure a hog could kill a horse.

You can see that the veterinarian does have to have a broader education then the human physician. Today he is getting it from the devoted faculty members who constitute the teaching profession.

Besides teaching their specialties, many faculty members conduct research. Just as in medical colleges, the professor is often expected to publish the results of his research and is frequently judged on the basis of such reports, so the veterinary faculty member is judged and promoted on the basis of his research.

There are several veterinary journals which are filled with research reports, many of them authored by veterinary college professors or other faculty members.

8

Other Important Areas of Involvement

Veterinarians in Quarantine and Inspection Work

When animals or birds are imported into the United States, some of the species must be quarantined for varying times in order that they not carry foreign diseases with them. All animals must be inspected by veterinarians at the ports of arrival. Dogs and cats are inspected, and if they appear to have no communicable or contagious diseases, are permitted to enter the country. Most of the other species such as circus animals, poultry, pigeons, farm animals, are taken to a quarantine station. A veterinarian inspects them at the pier and veterinarians in charge of the quarantine stations are constantly vigilant, watching for any outbreak of a disease. Rules are based on knowledge of diseases prevalent in exporting countries. For example, England may have an epizootic of foot-and-mouth disease. It is known that the virus is long-lived. So England may be embargoed because animals or birds from there could bring the virus to our country on their feet or in their hair or in the case of birds, on their feathers.

Results show that the quarantine service has indeed acted as a preventer of the spread of diseases, some of which could cost American agriculture large sums of money had the diseases swept through herds or flocks. Instead, the infected animals were detected at the quarantine stations and destroyed.

In addition to the quarantine veterinarians, a small but vital group of federal inspectors are concerned with the spread of established disease as well as being ever alert to the introduction of new diseases from avenues other than quarantine which could, if unchecked, reduce the flow of meat to a trickle in a few weeks in our country. The better the transportation facilities to move animals, the more potential danger to spread disease. We have the best transportation systems in the world. In an outbreak of a disease such as foot-and-mouth disease, animals would be shipped in haste by unscrupulous dealers and owners to avoid local quarantine and our meat production could be decimated in a short time.

As we said, federal veterinarians were sent to Mexico prior to 1954 and more recently to England to help with the control of outbreaks of foot-and-mouth disease in those countries. These men have invaluable experience for our protection. They have detailed plans of quarantine and slaughter should such an outbreak occur. With more and more animals being produced, the more devastating would be the results of such an outbreak.

Industrial Veterinarians

A growing field of veterinary endeavor is in industry. This is usually in a research capacity, but a goodly number of veterinarians are managers and officials in different branches of industry. Some have established and own veterinary pharmaceutical companies, some manufacture vaccines. The larger drug companies have veterinary divisions, each led by a graduate veterinarian. New drugs or biologics are tested to determine whether they will make worthwhile additions to the line of products marketed by the concern. Applications must be made to the Food and Drug Administration for permission to market these promising products, and they must be approved before they can be offered to the public.

Each application must be accompanied by reams of evidence indicating that the drug is safe and as efficacious as the manufacturer claims. Usually veterinarians must supervise the research.

The need for veterinarians in toxicology for industrial institutions is great, as all drugs used for man must first be proven nontoxic to lower animals.

Laboratory Animal Veterinarians

Many years ago as a busy practitioner, the senior author was invited to join the staff of the Yale Medical School to share his expertise a few times a year with those who were conducting research on lower animals, as well as to pursue research on his own. In those days, no veterinarians were trained in laboratory animal veterinary medicine.

Today, most medical schools have one, if not whole staffs of full-time veterinarians. Their functions are in research which they conduct with great effectiveness and service. The service consists of maintaining the health of research animal "colonies" as well as enforcing strict humane principles in caring for laboratory animals.

This is an area of great challenge since these professionals find problems never described before and work on new methods of diagnosis and treatment. If you would help mankind, here is one of the areas with the greatest potential for making a contribution to man's knowledge.

Zoo Veterinarians

Perhaps the most challenging and the most frustrating branch of veterinary medicine is the work of the zoo veterinarian.

There are no schools that teach zoo veterinary medicine in depth because the demand is so small. After all, how many zoos are there? How does one become a zoo veterinarian? Usually, a practitioner in a community is asked to help, on a part-time basis, with problems at the zoo. As the zoo grows, the veterinarian solves more and more problems and must spend more time until one day the zoo is large enough to require the full-time services of such a professional and the veterinarian is offered the job of zoo veterinarian. Some young veterinarians become apprentices to a veterinarian of long standing and take over one day.

We said it is most challenging and here's why. Trouble in the rodent house. The white-footed deer mice (one ounce) are sick and the peccary (100 pounds) isn't eating well. In the reptile house the growth in the Indian python's mouth must be removed. Someone fed the deer some chokecherry leaves through the fence, and the yellow-bellied sapsucker has a broken wing at the bird house. Nutrition, husbandry, injuries and disease, and then those visiting well-meaning dignitaries. Yes, it's challenging—but don't count on it, for there are so few possibilities.

Wildlife Veterinarians

A growing number of veterinarians are studying diseases of wildlife both in the wild and in captivity. Knowledge gained may be of greater importance to man himself than the species affected. Most of this work is done in universities.

Military Veterinarians

The Army and Air Force have their own veterinarians, about 800 in all. It is their duty to care for the animals of all kinds—horses, dogs and experimental species—under military supervision, as well as being concerned with the foods of animal origin used by the troops. They are Army and Air Force public health officials even though they have no public health degrees. In research they may be involved with chemical and bacteriological warfare.

When animals were sent into space flights, veterinarians studied the effects on these creatures, helping to determine the safety of the flights for the animals and for human beings who later followed them.

Sentry dogs, famous for their work during wartime, are maintained in good health by the military veterinarians.

Most importantly, the work of the Armed Forces veterinarians, in the field of food inspection, has been their chief contribution. They insure that all of the foods fed to troops are wholesome and safe and, in cooperation with food technologists, prepare the rations used in combat, in the form of dehydrated rations, precooked frozen meals, precooked meals, survival food packets and even food in liquid form.

Food and Drug Veterinarians

The Food and Drug Administration is thought of as testing the safety of products for human consumption but that is only part of the work of this great lifesaving institution; actually the veterinary or agricultural part of the FDA is extremely important. This is called the Bureau of Veterinary Medicine.

Manufacturers submit applications of new drugs for approval. One of the chief chores is passing on drugs which when added to animal feeds are supposed to increase growth rates. Over 7,000 applications for these substances were processed in 1969. This is important work. For example, if the

FDA approves the implantation of hormones into growing steers, will there be sufficient hormone residue left in the meat to have any effect on people who eat it?

Or, if hens are dewormed with a certain deworming drug of proved effectiveness, will the eggs from those hens be detrimental or retain the taste of the drug for a day or two following the deworming? If cows are treated for udder infections, will their milk be dangerous or taste from the drug? Such problems must be answered by FDA veterinarians before permission is granted to market drugs or methods. Sometimes several years are required to make such determinations. In one year well over 1,000 new drug applications are reviewed and their safety and efficacy determined by veterinarians.

Public Health

Virtually all veterinary medicine concerns itself with public health in the broad sense, such as the protection of the animals which must feed mankind and even the companion animals which are important to mental health. However, more specifically the public health veterinarian is concerned with over 150 zoonoses (diseases transmissible from lower animals to man). Constant control measures must be enforced and more research is imperative to answer so many unanswered questions concerning these diseases.

Many veterinarians obtain an additional degree in public health and are hired as public health veterinarians by the federal as well as municipal governments.

9

Three Typical Days in Practice

First, the large-animal practitioner. Living in a farming community where everybody is up early, our veterinarian is up early, too. No calls since ten last evening, he has had a sound night's sleep. Six A.M. finds him eating breakfast.

Three calls before 7:30 A.M., each from a farmer who needs assistance.

The doctor opens the back of his station wagon, already filled with drugs and equipment, fills his compact cooler (some have gas refrigerators built in) with ice cubes and puts in bottles of injectables which must be kept cool, picks up some sterile packs of surgical instruments and syringes, and, satisfied he has forgotten nothing, goes into the house for his several changes of uniforms and boots. He tests his intercom and with notebook beside him on the seat, is soon on his way to the first call. This one is only five miles out. He drives into the farmhouse yard, is invited in for coffee, refuses politely, slips on his special boots and with a syringe in one hand, a bottle of vaccine in the other, walks with his client toward a cattle chute. This is a long alley made of heavy planks nailed to strong posts. At one end is a stanchion. Into a large corral, a herd of over a hundred White Face cattle are milling about, unused to being confined in so small an area. Several boys and men are on hand. Their job is to keep the cattle moving through the chute and to operate the stanchion and heavy door.

The first steer gets his head into the stanchion and the boy atop the device pushes a 2 by 4 which holds the steer's head. The farmer pushes a bar across the chute behind the steer. The doctor injects the contents of the syringe under the skin of the animal. As he does so, he looks over the top plank and sees something of interest. Stepping up on a plank, he reaches over and runs his hand along the steer's back.

"Mr. Stephenson," he says, "are they all as bad as this?"

"Bad as what?" asks the farmer.

"Skin full of these bumps," the veterinarian answers. "These are cattle grubs. Better do something about them. Every one we kill means fewer next year."

"Didn't know they were this bad," the farmer says. "What have you got for them?"

"Paint their backs with insecticide or rub the dust in. Some will get into the openings and kill them but every one that comes out will get some on it and die."

The doctor goes to his car and returns with a large can.

"Here's some insecticide suspension. You paint every critter right now if you've got a big old paint brush." So Mr. Stephenson goes to a shed and returns with a new paint roller and pan.

"Great!" the doctor exclaims. Mr. Stephenson, sitting on

the top fence plank, rolls the toxic substance over the back of every steer as it is vaccinated and let out of the big door when the boy opens the stanchion.

And so the herd is protected against the dreaded disease, blackleg, against which only *protection,* not treatment, is the controlling factor. And now the cattle grubs which spoil cow hides and set the cattle back to some extent will not live to infest cattle next year.

The doctor changes his white coveralls, disinfects his boots and starts for the next call on his list. His intercom buzzes. His wife says, "Honey, go to the Jones's: something wrong with the family cow; acting strangely." He goes there before making his next scheduled call.

The Jones's cow is indeed acting strangely. The doctor smells her breath. She is tethered on a long chain held in place with a crowbar stuck into the ground.

"She hasn't been here all night, I'm sure," the doctor tells Mrs. Jones.

"No, doctor, we found her dragging the chain and staggering."

"I'll bet," the doctor replies. He sees a barrel under a tree; walks over and looks inside. It is a third full of apples and the surface of them is composed of partly chewed apples and slobber. He walks back to talk with Mrs. Jones.

"She's intoxicated, that's all," he says, and both have a laugh. "Was the barrel full of apples? She's made cider in her stomach, it fermented, and the alcohol's made her this way. I'll give her an injection to keep her quiet so she won't get up and stagger and maybe hurt herself. Sorry to have to charge you for telling you that you have a drunken cow. But she'll be all right as soon as she burns up the alcohol."

He goes to his next call where he vaccinates thirty pigs against hog cholera, the most dreaded affliction of all hog diseases. As he approaches his car, he hears his wife's voice. He picks up the receiver and listens. "The Bellow's colt is sick; kicked one side of the stall out. Better hurry. Only Ted is home and he's too young to handle it."

This calls for a long detour of fifteen miles. The colt is indeed sick. Now he is not kicking but lying in the stall, grunting with pain. It's really not a colt at all but now a grown three-year-old horse. Ted still thinks of it as a colt, however.

"Gosh," Ted says. "I don't want anything to happen to him now. Got him saddle-broke and he rides fine."

"Something already has happened to him," the doctor says. "You mean you don't want him to die. I don't think he will. But let's get those sharp ends of boards out of his way. He could thrash about and stick one into his side." So they tear out the rest of the flimsy partition, and get "The colt" on his feet and lead him out into the sunlight.

"First a tranquilizer," the doctor says. He injects a small amount of chemical into the horse's jugular vein. "Here, hold him, Ted," the doctor says passing the halter rope to the boy, and he goes to his car for the remedies and a stomach tube, a pump and a pail.

From a small vial he takes a drug and as he injects it, he explains. "This'll get his glands secreting and the juices will help cure the indigestion. Now he won't like this but he'll like it better than he would have if we hadn't given the tranquilizer first."

He pushes the rounded end of the stomach tube up one nostril until several feet have disappeared. Soon it is all the way to the animal's stomach. The other end is then attached to a pump and the solution is pumped into the animal. The tube is then removed.

"Now lead him around for half an hour, Ted, and phone me at home if he's not better by twelve thirty. I hope to make it by then, and tell your Dad to make the new partition of heavy planks, not boards. O.K.?"

He sets off for his next scheduled call.

Passing through town, the doctor stops to have lunch at a comfortable, homey restaurant where perhaps he eats roast beef from a local steer whose carcass he has inspected, since he is the local food inspector in addition to being a practitioner. Indeed, his next call is to inspect the carcass of a lamb which is to be delivered to this same restaurant.

The inspection over, the doctor, knowing the family is a large one, asks why the lamb was not cut up and frozen for the members of the family to eat. "Since it had been one of the family pets the children couldn't bear to eat it," the mother informs him.

Agreeing, and saying good-bye, he next goes to a dairy farm where he finds all the cows in their stanchions at 2:00 P.M. when normally they would not be in before 4:30 P.M. Here he starts the tuberculin test to try to discover any cattle harboring the disease. And here he especially needs his coveralls because he is working at the business end of the cow. A small syringe is filled from a vial. The needle is small because the biologic must be injected within the skin, not under it, and only a drop at that.

Quite rapidly the process is repeated on the over two hundred cows and young stock, faster indeed than one a minute.

In three days he must return and "read" the results of the test. If, on examination of the sites of injection, he finds a swelling, large or small, it is a certain revelation that that cow is a carrier of tuberculosis. He must condemn her for slaughter but the owner will be reimbursed for her value by the government.

By 4:00 P.M. the doctor heads for home and two appointments in his office. His wife tells him about two calls from farmers who have come for products they have had him purchase for them—products which they can administer themselves. One is a vitamin preparation to prevent moon blindness in the stockman's horses; the other, a special kind of deworming medicine for the rancher's sheep.

The doctor discusses the problems with his clients. One wants him to undertake contract work to look after his livestock, the other to ask about some work he can do to save himself a veterinarian's fee and spare the busy doctor from inconsequential efforts.

Now it is suppertime. The veterinarian thinks of *The Village Blacksmith* verse, "Something accomplished, something done, has earned a night's repose." But while he and his wife are watching their favorite television show, the phone rings.

"Yes, Willard, yes, Willard," he says. "I'll get there as fast as I can." This is a real emergency—the frequent nighttime complaint—"milk fever." And the cow trying to calve in the bargain. When the doctor enters the barn, he has a bottle of solution in one hand, the tube for administering it in the other, together with a bull lead. This last device is like a large pair of pincers, only the jaw is made with two rounded ends which fit one in each side of a critter's nose, and to the handle end, a rope is attached so that when it is in place, pulling on the rope keeps it there and the animal can be held.

The cow is lying on her chest and belly, head folded around to one side. The doctor inserts the bull lead into her nose. She is comatose and doesn't feel it. He inserts the needle into the jugular vein, connects the tube after he has attached the tube to the bottle and fills the tube by turning the bottle upside down. The farmer holds her head around so she can't attempt to rise. Finally the 500 cc. of solution is mixed with her blood and in a few minutes she appears normal and her body functions are no longer impaired.

Now for the calf. The cow can strain as her uterus contracts. She does and soon two front feet appear. The calf's nose can be seen between them. "Let's help her," the doctor suggests. "She's been through a lot and needs help. Besides, the calf may need to breathe. Let's hope it's alive."

The cow's head is pushed through the open stanchion by the client who locks her in. The doctor takes a firm hold on each of the calf's legs just above the joint and pulls. Each time the cow strains, he pulls. The head comes out. "Tongue's a little blue," the veterinarian states, "but I think we're in time." And just then the calf inspires one breath despite the pressure on its chest which is now passing through its mother's pelvis. More pulling and then, whoosh, the calf slides out and the doctor eases it down onto the straw which the farmer has spread behind her. The blueness leaves the tongue. The calf is lifted beside the dam and its mother's head is let out of the stanchion. She turns and licks the calf. After fifteen minutes, doctor and owner carry the calf to a box stall, the doctor goes to the house, washes, and this time not only has earned a night's repose but gets it.

And there you have a typical day in the life of a large-animal veterinarian, just one among days with endless variety.

A typical day in the life of a mixed-practice veterinarian might consist of the following: The doctor has a lively practice in the companion-animal field. His assistant, who is not a licensed veterinarian, takes care of such mundane chores as medicating dogs in the hospital according to the doctor's orders, answering the phone and keeping in touch with the doctor by intercom and making appointments. This doctor's schedule consists of outcalls in the morning, surgery late in the morning and late afternoon. The outcalls are usually on farm animals so, because farmers are early risers, the morning calls can start at 7:30 A.M.

This typical day opens with vaccination of a large herd of six-week-old pigs. The owner and his two sons have driven them into a small pen where they are packed together and easy to catch. The farmer sits on a chair. One son catches a pig, passes it over the fence to his brother who hands it to his father. The father holds the squealing pig upside down, belly toward the doctor who, quicker than we can write these words, has it vaccinated. Father turns the pig upright and the doctor pokes a deworming capsule, which he has inserted in the end of an instrument, down the pig's throat and the pig is turned loose. The job takes only an hour.

After answering some questions relating to other livestock, he removes his white coveralls, climbs into his car and starts for his next call. As he rides, he phones home base. No emergencies. So, on a farm five miles from the first, the doctor dons a clean uniform and boots, carries in his bag and a casting harness. This time his job is to castrate a fine quarter-horse colt, which he does with dispatch after the animal has been tranquilized and carefully restrained with ropes to prevent self-injury and injury to those managing the colt. The horse's head has rested on a bag of straw—its pillow—while the owner sits on his colt's head. The ropes are removed; the colt stands. Instructions for aftercare are given.

The next stop is at a farm where fine Angus cattle are raised. Eight cows are in the barn in stanchions. "They all failed to settle this spring," the owner tells the doctor. "Got to have a calf crop. Examine them and tell me whether to beef 'em or breed 'em again." Now the doctor wears only a pair of white pants. He strips down to his waist, washes, slips on a long sterile glove which reaches to his shoulder, reaches into the cow's rectum and through the walls he clearly feels the ovaries one at a time. The farmer takes notes of the veterinarian's findings.

"This one settled, but she's got a mummy in her. We'll fix that. She won't need to be beefed." The doctor removes a natural growth from the ovary.

He dons a new glove and feels in the next. "No reason this heifer didn't catch," he says. "Breed her again."

And so on. Only one he finds needs to be disposed of. But not the cow with the mummified fetus (a fairly common condition in cattle). She will pass it in four days.

So after washing and dressing, the doctor hies himself to his next call—a large show sow having trouble farrowing. She's so fat it is difficult to tell whether she has passed all her pigs. But because she seems content to lie without any seeming ambition, the owner is worried. "Gave her the medicine as you advised," the owner says. "Helped her for a while only." Into the pen both men climb; the doctor with his pig loop. First her temperature is taken. It is much too high. The huge sow seems oblivious to the ministrations of the men. The doctor diagnoses retained pigs or, anyway, placentas. He reaches his loop far up into the sow's uterus, hooks the end around a pig's neck and with a gentle pull, slowly removes it—a badly decomposed piglet. This large one has prevented the birth of several more. These in turn are pulled out and the last one is still alive. It gasps and breathes.

The old sow shows her relief, gets to her feet, drinks copiously, returns, grunts to the pigs and lies down again. The owner is even more relieved.

The intercom tells the doctor to hurry home; he has many operations awaiting his skill. So he arrives, cleans up, changes his shoes, dons his surgery gown and goes to work. Two ovariohysterectomies, a Caesarean section on a tiny Chihuahua, a broken leg set after an X-ray demonstrates the feasibility. A splint is bent into shape and applied to the anesthetized dog. It's lunchtime.

Afternoon office hours consist of a variety of ailments needing thoughtful consultation with the patients' owners. Vaccination of two Springers, a show cat to be examined for pregnancy so the owner who has sold it can guarantee to the new owner that her pet will have kittens; a parakeet, which swears at the doctor much to the owner's embarrassment, has an abnormal lump on one wing (it is scheduled for surgery the following day); a Beagle whose rear is peppered with bird shot, some of which are removed in a time-consuming operation; the tip of a Foxhound's ear to be sutured to stop slow bleeding; six baby skunks to be descented. This last job, the doctor explains, he can't do until all the rest of the day's work is done. (Some states require a permit to keep wild animals.)

Next is the fancier with a box containing eight fancy pigeons—Jacobins—which he wants to send to Canada. The birds are examined, health forms filled out which the doctor must send for government approval, and that call is completed.

More operations. The six skunks descented. The doctor thinks he had done it odorlessly but his wife at supper comes to the table, a clothespin clasped on her nose. They both laugh; it is her way of notifying her husband that he missed, ever so little.

A shower is in order and the doctor goes back to evening office hours. A light evening interrupted with a few phone calls. Come 10:00 P.M., bed feels fine.

And lastly, a day in a busy small-animal veterinary hospital. This being one of our own which we chose after looking back over the diary to pick one of the more interesting with considerable variety. At the time, there were three of us veterinarians working in the clinic, and it was Dr. Leon's duty to perform most of the surgery.

Many veterinarians operating their own practices see clients only by appointment and operate all morning if there are sufficient operations on the list. Some days one of us operated all day long but on this day only the morning was so occupied; the other two men were seeing the clients.

The operations began at 8:00 A.M. An assistant had sterilized ten sets of instruments, drapes and rubber gloves, which he knew, from having read the schedule, would be needed. There were seven ovariohysterectomies (spay operations). As these were uncomplicated short operations, an injectable anesthetic was used. A nurse kept the animals under observation while in the recovery room.

Now came an English Setter with a huge lump in her abdomen. We all thought the dog was a hopeless case. After putting her on the gas machine for general anesthesia, scrubbing, prepping and draping the site, a long incision was made on her midline and the tumor exposed. The incision had to be lengthened to allow for passage of the cancer which was growing in the spleen. The spleen was removed, the tumor—the size of a large grapefruit—with it, and the incision closed. The operation was successful and the owner was made a happy man, for the Setter was an outstanding hunter. Time of operation, ninety minutes.

A Great Dane returned home limping. X-ray indicated a broken leg and this operation entailed building an aluminum splint adjusted to hold it in place, and re-X-raying to be sure the final alignment was perfect. Now it was lunchtime.

Afternoon consisted of a Caesarean operation and attending to clients' animals. The first client had a huge coonhound he had just bought. From its mouth came a truly obnoxious odor, and it was obviously in pain. An emetic was in order. The owner was asked to take him outside where he vomited part of a young skunk and some garbage he had also eaten.

The receptionist hurried out to tell us there was an emergency. We found an Airedale in the arms of his owner and the cause of the dog's trouble was visible! He had attacked a porcupine and was badly quilled. One side had no quills but the other entire shoulder and front leg was white with the ends of small tail quills. And the face was bristling with them.

We reached for the anesthetic to stop all muscle movement and lay the dog on the examining table. Giving an assistant a pair of strong forceps, we both pulled quills as fast as we could. Some, of course, broke off and many had already moved in out of sight. None was in the rib cage so we could predict that we could save the dog. Even the tongue, the lips and palate were bristling. But after two hours we had removed every quill except those gone out of sight in the shoulder. We told the owner he would start to feel the quills coming out above the shoulder blades in a few days, loaned him forceps and explained that the points would be easy to pull out.

A horn tooted and the receptionist went out where a man was sitting in a car and attempting to hold a large ewe on the floor beside him. We were appraised and together we carried the poor thing to the operating room. A large flap of skin had been torn loose by a dog. Its tail was only a red stump with all the skin gone from it. This animal was in shock.

"Pet?" we asked.

"Not especially," he replied.

"Then I'd kill her and collect from the state," we replied.

"Can't," he said, " 'cause if I do, my neighbor's dog will have to be killed. That's the law, isn't it? But why kill her?"

"Because a ewe run and then attacked by dogs is seldom worth anything," We told him. "We'll sew her up if you want but she'll be better off dead."

"How much to kill her?"

"Office call and another charge to cremate."

"Go ahead. I'll bury her and save the cremation charge."

That was that and we changed our coats because a sheep held in one's arms makes one smell like a sheep.

The Caesarean had to be done. We delivered a nice litter of Boston Terriers.

The last client before supper had a tomcat with a urinary stoppage. It had to be relieved or it would die of uremic poisoning. The strong urine was removed with a catheter after the minute crystalline deposits had been displaced. We were leaving for home when in drove a man with two litters of Springer Spaniels needing vaccination. This didn't take long and they were on their way with a warning to the owner to keep them away from all strange dogs for a week until immunity could begin to develop.

And so to supper. Another average day except that two days each week one of us returned and worked until the last client had gone, which was often eleven o'clock at night. The other men worked the other four evenings.

So now we're sure you believe what we said at the beginning: we are not acting as missionaries to lure you into our profession. No, we're giving you an honest picture of it as it really is. We have chosen typical examples of what you may expect if, as we hope, you become a veterinarian.

10

Have You Got What It Takes?

What does it take, in the way of mental and physical qualifications, to be a successful veterinarian? You have been given a brief look at the divisions of the profession, and have read descriptions of three typical days in lives of practitioners. You can pretty much decide for yourself whether or not you have the strength, endurance, and mental ability for whatever branch you want to enter.

Almost certainly you have what it takes if you want it badly enough. Yes, you have, because as you have seen, there are so many kinds of work in the various fields of veterinary medicine. We assume that you have an interest or you wouldn't have read this book, so it comes down to a matter of energy. Energy in turn, depends on physique and the dynamo within each of us which keeps us ticking. We said *almost certainly*. The *almost* refers to moral courage and that we shall deal with later.

Manifestly, there are those in any profession whose supply of energy is not of the order which drives a man or woman to great achievement. And, contrariwise, there are those whose drive, and the ability and physical resources to sustain it, make leisure almost obnoxious.

Those with a weak drive who feel the need of leisure can find a niche in veterinary medicine; those average persons who can "stand the gaff" but who often feel the need for rest can find a place too. Those whose gadflies of ambition and drive keep them "everlastingly at it" will find a welcome in areas which demand strength and endurance, areas such as the large-animal field, or even the small-animal if it is a busy practice. Such a person seems to attract clients, and makes of his practice an active success.

You may start out in one field, find it not to your liking, and change to another. Many a practitioner is today teaching in a veterinary medical college. Others have quit their practices to become pathologists, research workers and, not infrequently, food inspectors. There are many examples of such changes. For one, men have given up active practices, gone back to college, taken advanced courses in pathology and are now animal pathologists in large universities. Others, who were appointed while practicing to the city health commissions, decide their contribution to public health could be of more value to society and more to their liking. They go back to college for two years and become doctors of public health, in addition to being veterinarians.

Still others, after graduation, successfully pass the state board examinations, work in a busy veterinary hospital for six months and decide by then "I've had it; too demanding for me." They may accept excellent positions in research with pharmaceutical companies.

Moving in the opposite direction, one finds men who are

not content with the smaller salaries of the food inspector, researcher, teacher, who have abundant energy and who leave the relative security of these branches of the profession to establish practices. Some veterinarians move in this direction every year, but the number is not nearly as great as those who move to jobs requiring less energy.

Don't think you will be making all the decisions after your marriage; your wife will indeed have a considerable influence on your future. And so may your children.

The ideal human being has been described as the intelligent, adaptable, good sport with a sense of humor. It takes considerable adaptability to cope with unexpected changes. And good sportsmanship to keep up with them. If you have these qualities, you can surmount any changes which occur in your future and still stay within the framework of veterinary medicine.

But depending on your age, perhaps it is not a good idea to make up your mind what your specialty shall be if you haven't even entered college. Young people learn a lot and change a lot—then ideas change too. One unreasonable professor in a college subject can make that really highly interesting subject almost repulsive; a different professor might have made it so attractive that many students would decide to follow it as their life's work.

This is our advice if you decide to be a veterinarian: make that decision but decide on your specialty *after* you get to college. Picture yourself a full-fledged veterinarian, and hold such a mental image with all your aspirations and hopes met. It will help you to attain it.

11

Your Education

The shortest distance between two points is a straight line. Any truly successful man will tell you that in order to achieve success, in the shortest possible time, one needs a goal. In your case perhaps you already have the goal, namely, to become a veterinarian. And so you want to attain that goal in the shortest possible time and be thoroughly prepared to assume what responsibilities are necessary while you are achieving it.

In the case of some men and women, it is sometimes necessary to take a circuitous route in order to reach the goal of becoming a veterinarian. We could state many instances, some almost tragic, to illustrate this point. Unfortunately, young men and women find that they have to take an extra year of high school because they weren't careful enough to chart their course in advance along that straight line. Sometimes the wrong course in high school is followed instead of a college preparatory course.

If you are aware that you would like to make your life goal in the field of veterinary medicine before you are through your first year in high school, you should write to all the veterinary colleges in which you might be accepted. You won't be acceptable to many because of the place you live. Naturally, each veterinary college must have a limitation on the number of students it enrolls. This number usually varies from forty to one hundred and twenty five a year so that obviously if five hundred New York City men and women applied to Cornell University, there would not be room for all of them. On the other hand, the state of California did not establish its veterinary college to educate people from New York State. Rightfully, each state that has a veterinary college considers that it is supporting its college for the benefit of its own agriculture and the benefit of its own citizens. Its first choice, therefore, must be the students from its own state. However, in order to save money and avoid the necessity of establishing veterinary colleges in every state, some states have made agreements with others enabling them to send some of their students to the neighboring states which do have veterinary colleges. And so an agreement was reached as to the geographical regions from which each college would accept applicants. This is sensible because each section has its own more or less specific problems. The cattle of some areas tend to be dairy types, those in others, beef. In the densely populated areas, there will be more companion animals.

Here is an alphabetical list of our nation's veterinary schools and the areas from which they are willing to accept applications. It will save you time sending for catalogues because the restrictions are the word of the deans of whom we asked this specific information.

Auburn University, School of Veterinary Medicine, Auburn, Alabama 36830: Admissions restricted to residents of the states in this area. One hundred and five students were admitted in 1970.

Colorado State University, College of Veterinary Medicine and Biomedical Sciences, Fort Collins, Colorado 80521: Accommodated eighty-four students in the freshman class in 1970 in the following order of preference: 1) Colorado residents, 2) Students from the Western Interstate Commission for Higher Education and Nebraska, and 3) Students from other states and foreign countries.

Iowa State University, College of Veterinary Medicine, Ames, Iowa 50010: Iowa State considers applications from students residing in any of the United States. Preference is given to those who are residents of Iowa. There were eighty students in the 1970 freshman class.

Kansas State University, College of Veterinary Medicine, Manhattan, Kansas 66502: When a class is selected for admission the best-qualified Kansas students are chosen first; then if class positions remain, the applicants from states without veterinary colleges are selected; and finally (rarely) those from states with veterinary colleges are considered. Only eighty-five students in the freshman class were admitted in 1970.

Michigan State University, College of Veterinary Medicine, East Lansing, Michigan 48823: Michigan State will accept well-qualified students from any state. First priority for admission is given to Michigan residents. The vast majority of the nonresident students have been Michigan State University preveterinary students. There were one hundred and five students admitted in the freshman class in 1970.

New York State Veterinary College at Cornell University, Ithaca, New York 14850: New York State Veterinary College now accepts forty-five students from New York State and twenty from elsewhere. Preference is given to applicants from the New England area and to applicants from states which have no veterinary school.

Ohio State University, College of Veterinary Medicine, Columbus, Ohio 43210: Applications are accepted from highly qualified students from all states. Education agreements have been established with the following states: West Virginia, Kentucky, Florida, Oregon, Maryland. Under the terms of the agreements six students who are considered competitive are considered for admission. One hundred and twenty students were accepted in the 1970 freshman class.

Oklahoma State University, College of Veterinary Medicine, Stillwater, Oklahoma 74074: 1) Oklahoma residents are given preference, 2) Certified residents of states under contract agreement from West Virginia, North Carolina, Louisiana, Arkansas, North Dakota, and Nebraska are considered, 3) Students are accepted from states which have no veterinary school, and 4) Applications are accepted from students of other states and foreign countries. Forty-nine students were accepted in the 1970 freshman class.

Purdue University, School of Veterinary Medicine, Lafayette, Indiana 47907: Applications of students who are residents of Indiana are given first consideration, second consideration is given to applicants from states that do not have a veterinary college or a regional pact with a veterinary college, and third consideration is given to those candidates from states that do have a veterinary college. These are basic guidelines. The admissions committee is quite interested in a student's overall academic record and other items that can be gleaned from the application. Sixty-five students were accepted in the 1970 freshman class.

Texas A&M University, College of Veterinary Medicine, College Station, Texas 77843: The order of priority is: Applications accepted from Texas residents and contract states and foreign countries with interinstitutional contracts, from states and foreign countries with no veterinary schools, and from other states with veterinary schools. The student body is comprised of students from Texas and Louisiana due to this priority system. There were one hundred and twenty-eight in the 1970 freshman class, the largest number of the eighteen schools.

Tuskegee Institute, School of Veterinary Medicine, Tuskegee, Alabama 36088: Tuskegee Institute accepts students from any state. It does have definite contract quotas with states in the Southern Regional Educational Board. These states are: Florida, South Carolina, North Carolina, Virginia, West Virginia, Maryland, Kentucky, Tennessee, Georgia, Mississippi, and Louisiana. The student body generally consists of students from over two dozen states, Puerto Rico, the District of Columbia and several foreign countries. Thirty-nine students were accepted in the 1970 freshman class.

University of California, School of Veterinary Medicine, Davis, California 95616: Applications are accepted in the following order from students from all states and from any foreign country: California residents, students from states affiliated with the Western Interstate Commission for Higher Education, students from states with no veterinary school and students from states that have a veterinary school. There were eighty-five students admitted in the 1970 freshman class.

University of Georgia, School of Veterinary Medicine, Athens, Georgia 30601: Applications for admission are accepted from all states and countries but preferential consideration is given to residents of Georgia, Maryland, North Carolina, South Carolina and Virginia. There were sixty-nine students admitted in the 1970 freshman class.

University of Illinois, College of Veterinary Medicine, Urbana, Illinois 61801: Preference is given to Illinois residents. Each year a few outstanding students are accepted from states which do not presently support a professional school of their own. There were seventy-eight students admitted in the 1970 freshman class.

University of Minnesota, College of Veterinary Medicine, St. Paul, Minnesota 55101: Sixty students are accepted each year in the first year class. Preference is given to residents of Minnesota and the economic area not having a professional school (i.e., North Dakota, South Dakota and Wisconsin). There were sixty-six students admitted in the freshman class of 1970.

University of Missouri, School of Veterinary Medicine, Columbia, Missouri 65201: There are no restrictions concerning states from which students are accepted. However, higher priority is given to students from states without schools of veterinary medicine. There were sixty-five students admitted in the 1970 freshman class.

University of Pennsylvania, School of Veterinary Medicine, Philadelphia, Pennsylvania 19104: Qualified applicants from all fifty states, as well as students from foreign countries are accepted. However, preference is given to Pennsylvania residents. There were eighty-two students admitted in the 1970 freshman class. The percentage of women students admitted is higher than for any other school.

Washington State University, College of Veterinary Medicine, Pullman, Washington 99163: Students from all states are accepted according to the following priority system: 1) Washington residents, 2) Residents of states of their regional compact (Oregon, Idaho, Montana, Utah, Nevada, New Mexico, Arizona, Hawaii and Alaska), and 3) The remainder of the applicants from the remaining states. There were sixty students admitted to the 1970 freshman class.

Assuming that you have written to the dean of admissions of each of the veterinary colleges to which you wish to apply, you open the catalogue to entrance requirements and from this, chart your high school courses. It might be beneficial for you to see the principal or guidance counselor of your high school and explain your ambition and tell him why you are taking the courses upon which you have decided. We strongly urge that you do not neglect taking as many English courses as you can. Learn speed reading. Remember that one thinks with words. Our impression is that most of the veterinarians with whom we were educated took the minimum number of English courses because they felt it required too much outside reading. It does, but if you train yourself to read reasonably fast, you will have no trouble on that account and your education will be better rounded.

Before one is accepted into any of the colleges of veterinary medicine, some preliminary college education is required. In most of the colleges, two or three years of preveterinary education are demanded. The courses in preveterinary medicine are usually identical to the courses in premedicine, and so you will be studying with students who plan to go on to human medicine. Many students have attended the state university in their state, and after the second year apply to a veterinary school in another state which they wish to attend. They are usually not accepted. Again, after the third year the chances are much better of being accepted but many find that it is necessary to go for four years in preveterinary medicine before they can be accepted in the veterinary school. You should plan to take at least three years, and then, if your grades are high enough, your other credentials such as exposure to the profession in a veterinary hospital or working on a farm or both will enhance your chances for acceptance. In all of the schools of veterinary medicine may be found students who have already obtained advanced degrees and therefore the average number of preveterinary years in many of the veterinary institutions is 3.9. Although the minimum number of years listed in the catalogues for most schools is two years of preveterinary work, it is rare that a student gains admission on this basis since there are so many applicants with more than two years of preveterinary work applying.

Preveterinary studies may be carried out in any accredited college, although there seems to be a better chance of being accepted when that education is in the same institution as the veterinary college. There are a limited number of places to be filled, so the student needs a high average to gain admittance. Usually a student will need a "B" average or better to be accepted.

The curriculum for preveterinary courses differs from one college or university to another, so it behooves a prospective student to send to the institution of his choice for the correct requirements in order to be prepared. Even while a junior in high school, some flexibility of choice is possible which will make the preveterinary courses easier. For example, one reads that biology is a required course in college, so if one takes biology in his senior year in high school, the college course will be easier and a higher grade can be expected.

Applicants for acceptance into most of the veterinary colleges should include the following:

1. An application form properly filled out.
2. An official transcript from the college or university attended sent directly from the dean of that institution.
3. A list of courses in which the applicant is enrolled or plans to become enrolled.
4. A copy of a physical examination report signed by a physician.
5. A recent photograph of the applicant.

6. Check or money order for the application fee, which is usually higher for out-of-state students.

7. Score records for any special tests or measurements, such as school or college ability tests.

8. As many recommendations from leading citizens and alumni as possible.

Each veterinary college sets its own time (usually about March 1) for completion of the application, to receive consideration for admission to the class entering in September of the same year.

We can't emphasize enough that the veterinary colleges were not organized to educate veterinarians to take care of companion animals. You must find out from the veterinary school in which you hope to matriculate how important this is, for there are indications at this time that some of the institutions are relaxing their farm experience requirements.

With this step behind us, now what about veterinary education? Although the courses are standard courses in all of the colleges, the depth of study often varies. Several of our friends who were not able to gain admission to American colleges, enrolled in foreign schools. Some have been graduated from Sidney, Australia; many have obtained their degrees from French and German schools.

Here is a list of subjects you may expect to cover during the four years of veterinary education. Many are so basic that students studying human medicine, dentistry, and other disciplines may take the same courses.

SAMPLE CURRICULUM OF A U.S. VETERINARY COLLEGE

FIRST YEAR

Gross Anatomy of Domestic Animals
Neuroanatomy

Histology and Embryology
Animal Husbandry
Physiological Chemistry
Physiology
Animal Genetics
Botany

SECOND YEAR

Radiobiology
Physiology
Experimental Physiology
Bacteriology and Immunology Laboratory
General Pathology
General Pathology Laboratory
Special Pathology
Special Pathology Laboratory
Parasitology
Animal Husbandry
Pharmacology
Public Health

THIRD YEAR

Public Health and Preventive Medicine
General Surgery
Surgical Exercises
Non-Infectious Diseases
Infectious Diseases of Large Animals
Small-Animal Medicine
Small-Animal Surgery
Applied Anatomy
Obstetrics
Clinical Pathology
Special Surgery
Diseases of Poultry
Roentgenology

FOURTH YEAR

Large-Animal Surgery
Small-Animal Surgery
Special Pathology
Jurisprudence, Ethics, and Business Methods
Clinical Conferences
Clinics
Laboratory-Animal Medicine
Toxicology
Nutrition

Cost of a Veterinary Education

The catalogue of the college of your choice will inform you of the current expenses of attending both the preveterinary and the professional course. There is no standard rate of fees, nor any standard for out-of-state charges. As an illustration, the fees at Purdue are (in 1971) $820 a year for Indiana residents and the nonresidents must pay $905 additional. Cornell charges $825 for New York State residents and $1,225 for nonresidents. Pennsylvania charges $1,950 for in-state students and $2,550 for out-of-state students.

In some states the overall college expenses are considerably less than in others, due principally to fees for room and board. The total expenses, excluding tuition, will run to approximately $2,500 a year including transportation, and expenses from unexpected incidentals. In some colleges there are opportunities to earn money in the latter years of the course, but it is not advisable to start college with that in mind; it is probably better to remain out of college and earn money for a year and save one's self worry. College should be a period in one's life when happy memories accumulate. Being constantly plagued with money worries not only reduces the chances of happy memories but cuts down on high achievement because attention must be given to earning money instead of learning.

Veterinary students are advised to work on farms or in hospitals during the summer vacations where the pay is low for such temporary employment. These students could earn more in other occupations but they gain more in the long run even though they do not save as much money as they might if they worked at other jobs.

Scholarships are available in most colleges for outstanding students. Banks or other institutions will loan money, especially when the student can obtain endorsement from financially responsible persons. Check into National Health Professions Student Loans, National Defense Student Loans, University Loans and G.I. Loans.

12

The State Board Examinations

You have completed your college course, been graduated and are the proud possessor of a certificate which says you have earned a veterinary degree.

But you are not yet a practicing veterinarian. That you cannot be until you have taken and satisfactorily passed a state board examination. This is offered to qualified men, usually twice a year. In the past, one requirement, no longer necessary, was that a veterinarian had to be graduated from a school accredited by the American Veterinary Medical Association. Since it is not possible to accredit each school in the world on a yearly basis, this requirement has been eliminated. A group—the state board of examiners—may require your passing a national board examination or compose the examination itself which is different in each of the states and changes with each examination. Usually an oral practical exam is also given. And these exams should be different, obviously, because the problems of a veterinarian in Florida would naturally be somewhat different from those in Oregon. Livestock parasite problems are of paramount importance to Floridians because of the lack of cold winter which Wisconsin has to decrease the ravages of parasites. New York, with its high concentration of human beings in cities, should ask more questions about companion animals than Wyoming where livestock is so important. Veterinarians practicing in a great sheep-growing state should know more about sheep than those practicing in primarily cattle-growing states.

So you decide where you want to practice, if practicing is the branch of veterinary medicine which interests you most, and you pay the fee and register to take the examination.

We strongly advise that you take as many examinations in states in which you might like to practice as you possibly can because the information which you need to have to pass many examinations will be fresh in your memory. The examinations will be general. We doubt many practitioners ten years out of college could pass the written exams of most states.

You must remember that no state wants too many animal doctors. We think of Florida, a glorious state to which many an elderly veterinarian would enjoy retiring and operating a nice leisurely practice during the tourist season. If Florida has no way of restricting the number of practicing veterinarians, there might soon be an overabundance. When that occurs, it results either in price cutting, which is harmful to the profession, or price fixing, which is detrimental to the public, and illegal.

On the other hand, there are states where there is a dearth of veterinarians. There are areas where two may be as many as a hundred miles apart. In such states, almost everyone passes the state boards.

One of the best indications of how badly veterinarians are needed in the United States is the number of candidates who take and the number who pass the tests.

The records indicate that in the areas of highest human population a smaller percent of candidates taking the examinations pass. And conversely, in those states with the smallest human population there is a larger percentage of candidates passing. Besides this knowledge, there are some other facts you should know which may help you to pass.

First, live up to the letter of the rules while you are waiting to take the exam. Suppose you take a job as an assistant to an established veterinarian. You work for him, five months, and in your spare time review your college studies. The rules of the State Veterinary Association allow this provided you do not operate or prescribe. Then your boss becomes sick. He tells you to do some operations for him, regardless of the rules. You do. Word gets to a member of the state board. Do you think that would enhance your chances of passing the exam? If your marks are equal to those of a man who has lived up to the letter of the law, he will be the one chosen first, assuming of course the board feels there are only a given number to be passed.

It is usually possible to obtain copies of examinations which have been given previously. When Dr. Leon took New York State exams, he learned that the Cornell senior class had been drilled in answering questions which had been given over the previous five years. This gave the graduates a big advantage. Such questions should be obtained wherever possible because they give the candidate an inkling of what kinds of questions he may be called on to answer.

Someday, perhaps by the time you who read this book and have been graduated from college, a national board exam will be given and passing it will entitle you to practice in any state in the Union. There is a national board exam now which all graduates may take if they desire, but this does not qualify one for practicing. Unless the jealous guardianship which some state boards exercise today is greatly changed, this is hardly to be expected for many years to come.

13

Getting Established

At the time of this writing the eighteen schools in the United States average about 5.6 jobs available to each graduate.

If you have decided to become a research veterinarian or a government employee before you are out of college, many opportunities will be open upon graduation. You will have been appraised of them in your senior year. Some of the larger commercial companies may send representatives to meet the seniors and discuss employment. But what about you who have decided to practice?

In your steps toward your goal, you have now passed your state board exams and are entitled to set up your practice anywhere you wish within that state. If you have decided on a large-animal practice, finding a location is easy compared with finding one on which to build a small-animal hospital.

Country towns or cities in sparsely settled states present

few obstacles. One can almost always find a desirable location on the outskirts of such a city. Not so with surburban districts in heavily populated states. Zoning laws prohibit the establishment of veterinary hospitals anywhere except in areas zoned for business. Even there, neighbors located in adjoining zones may object to kennel runs being erected because they know how dogs can upset their serenity by barking. So it becomes necessary to establish beyond the suburbs. But this is often advantageous because once established, the growing suburb cannot force the relocation of the hospital if and when that suburb catches up and surrounds the veterinary institution.

To become established as a general practitioner costs only a fraction of what it does to become a small-animal practitioner. And many of the general practitioners begin modestly. Many of them build a small building and install some cages even in their garages to take care of small animals. Some of the busiest large-animal men in America work out of their homes and vans. Some use their own airplanes in making calls.

So you see, it does not necessarily cost very much to get started in this way. What one needs is an office and someone to answer the telephone. That person might even assist at surgery. You must have an automobile; and an intercom system from the car to the home is practically a necessity today, although it is possible to start without one. There was a time when every veterinarian returned home after each call: today it's different. The receptionist or secretary who answers the telephone turns on the intercom system and speaks to the veterinarian in his car or wherever he may be and tells him where the next call is to be made. Thus, he becomes a much more efficient person. For the country veterinarian, these small and large animal practices can be mixed quite well and no one takes offense when the veterinarian returns from having taken care of hogs and perhaps can't shake off all of the hog odor. But where the veterinarian is a suburbanite or a city man, the two do not mix well at all.

Where is the money coming from to get established? There are several ways of obtaining it. One is to work for another large-animal veterinarian and it is nearly always a simple matter to find one who needs an assistant. He will probably make you sign an agreement that you will not practice within a given number of miles of his practice if he takes you in as an assistant and shows you his methods. This is only fair and right. Another way is to borrow the money from a bank, but this means that someone must sign the note as collateral. And, of course, another way is to simply start on plain old-fashioned nerve. Companies which sell drugs and instruments will often stake a veterinarian to several hundred dollars credit to help him get started in the hope and expectancy that he will remain loyal to that concern and buy drugs and instruments from them in the future. Some large-animal veterinarians have a good-sized dispensary of their own and dispense their own drugs while others write prescriptions. Most farmers prefer veterinarians to bring the medicines with them and leave them to use when further treatment is necessary.

Another way of getting started is to buy an already established practice; in that case one need not worry about location. But this can be an expensive proposition. Sometimes elderly veterinarians will sell a half-interest, agreeing to retire and sell the other half for an agreed price in a given number of years. During your practice with him, you learn many useful facts from your partner and better still become acquainted with his clients.

The location you choose in which to practice will depend, of course, upon the kind of practice you want, the number of established veterinarians and perhaps the prosperity of the area.

Michigan has a placement service and other states will probably follow by establishing these services to show veterinarians the areas where they are needed. By using large maps which show the density of population and the number of head of livestock, and the location of practicing veterinarians, the need is made quite clear.

The Michigan service was started, naturally, for the senior students of Michigan State University. Each of them fills out a form which advises the council of the area which most interests him and the type of practice he wants to follow. The council recommends a community for each student and supplies a roster of all the interesting facts about that community, supplies the names of professional men and public officials whom the student can contact and suggests a visit to the town or city. Every large area has a veterinary adviser whom the student can also contact.

This service is not now limited to Michigan students; the state needs veterinarians and any graduate or senior in the veterinary school may register and obtain the service.

In the event you are interested in the income you can earn —and who isn't?—we can tell you that it runs about equal to that of a comparable physician. Some men who own hospitals have an annual net income of over $50,000. The same man, when starting his practice, may have earned a gross of perhaps $10,000 but in a few years earned a net of $10,000 to $20,000 a year.

The same scale of salary holds for reseachers as for other biologists. The salary of food inspectors begins at about $8,-

000 and runs to well over $15,000. The government has increased salaries as the cost of living index increased. Here the fringe benefits in paid vacations, insurance and retirement plans are attractive.

14

The Future of Veterinary Medicine

There is little doubt that veterinary medicine has one of the brightest futures of any profession today. The fact that there are about six jobs available to each graduate in the United States as depicted to us by the deans of the eighteen schools, is a good indication of a great demand at this time for those professional people. And at a time when many endeavors are cutting back, the veterinary profession is leaping forward.

If you are interested in the opportunity to contribute a great deal to your society, this may be the profession for you.

At this time, one new veterinary school is accepting applications. Louisiana State University will graduate its first class in five years. Florida has drawing-board plans for a school of veterinary medicine and the New England Board of Higher Education has been charged by the governors of the New Enggland states to study the feasability and location for a school in the Northeast.

Most of the schools in existence have plans for a yearly increase in admissions. Even with the accomplishment of the most ambitious plans, there will continue to be a dire shortage in almost all fields of veterinary science. The research in problems in lower animals which also affect man is so vast that it is almost limitless.

The ecological problems in lower animals may well be the most important facing the veterinary profession and perhaps mankind.

The great advances in medicine are seldom appreciated by people today because so few remember how different things were when we didn't have all the new life-saving drugs and surgical techniques. The veterinarian will continue to contribute to the development of new and more wonderful life-saving drugs and better surgical techniques, not only for the welfare of lower animals but also directly applicable to use in man.

Will veterinary medicine in practice become, like human medicine, a profession of specialists? Will there be surgeons, skin specialists, cancer specialists, dieticians, pediatricians and so on? The answer is almost certainly "yes." Even at this time we have specialists in most of the fields of veterinary medicine in the veterinary universities of the land, and many are coming to the fore in private practice. At the moment, some are considered to be specialists in quite broad fields and therefore they are not specialists at all—for example, the horse specialist or the canine specialist.

As our population continues to expand, more and more food is needed. More milk for children, more meat for all. And as the human food supply runs ever closer to the point where human starvation begins, the efficiency of meat and milk production becomes increasingly more imperative. The cow which on the same food produces 6,000 quarts of milk a year as the cow which produces 18,000, must go. The sheep which grows four pounds of wool a year when other sheep can produce twelve, must disappear. The beef cattle which grow to 600 pounds in even a month longer than others, will have to be replaced. Parasites must be drastically reduced. The local veterinarian must, in the future, become more involved with genetics and nutrition, as well as being a doctor of diseases and surgery. He will become more and more respected as a member in every community.

Society is embarked on programs of combatting environmental pollution before it affects man. The veterinary profession must play a leading role here since it is the only group of educated and aware professionals ready to recognize the problems of lower animals brought about by pollution. In recognizing some of these problems, the profession may well be able to save some of the endangered species on earth—including man. For virtually every human malady there is a model lower animal with a similar problem. It is through investigations of lower animals that we find the answers to these problems, and these answers have in the past and will in the future be of great benefit to mankind. The veterinarian is the one person most qualified to study the ailments of lower animals, with his training in the abnormal as well as the normal of each species.

Ever-increasing numbers of veterinarians will find positions in medical schools to aid in the research of lower animals. More and more veterinarians will be courted to take their part in the work done in investigations of new drugs by the great drug companies of the country, and more and more will be needed by the Federal Government to test and verify the effects of the products submitted to them for approval by the drug companies. More and more will be necessary to watch over the ever-increasing food supplies to see to it that disease is not spread by way of the food which will be required in larger and larger amounts. With the constantly increasing horse population, more and more equine-oriented veterinarians will be needed to care for these animals.

A whole new field may soon be developed by the profession, and that is in oceanographic veterinary medicine, one of the woefully neglected areas of lower-animal maladies.

Considering the small supply and the great demand, the variety of opportunities open, and the challenges of the moment and the future, the horizons for a career in veterinary medicine are very bright.